LEADERSHIP
IN
HEALTHCARE

D0913261

LEADERSHIP IN HEALTHCARE

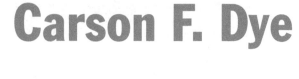

Essential Values and Skills

THIRD EDITION

Carson F. Dye

ACHE Management Series

Your board, staff, or clients may also benefit from this book's insight. For more information on quantity discounts, contact the Health Administration Press Marketing Manager at (312) 424–9450.

This publication is intended to provide accurate and authoritative information in regard to the subject matter covered. It is sold, or otherwise provided, with the understanding that the publisher is not engaged in rendering professional services. If professional advice or other expert assistance is required, the services of a competent professional should be sought.

The statements and opinions contained in this book are strictly those of the author(s) and do not represent the official positions of the American College of Healthcare Executives or the Foundation of the American College of Healthcare Executives.

21   5   4

Library of Congress Cataloging-in-Publication Data
Names: Dye, Carson F., author.
Title: Leadership in healthcare : essential values and skills / Carson F. Dye.
Other titles: Leadership in health care
Description: Third edition. | Chicago, IL : Health Administration Press, [2017] |
    Series: ACHE management series | Includes bibliographic references and index.
Identifiers: LCCN 2016027212 (print) | LCCN 2016028074 (ebook) | ISBN 9781567938463
    (alk. paper) | ISBN 9781567938470 (Ebook) | ISBN 9781567938487 (Xml) | ISBN
    9781567938494 (Epub) | ISBN 9781567938500 (Mobi)
Subjects: LCSH: Health services administration. | Leadership.
Classification: LCC RA971 .D937 2017 (print) | LCC RA971 (ebook) | DDC 362.1068/4–dc23
LC record available at https://lccn.loc.gov/2016027212

The paper used in this publication meets the minimum requirements of American National Standard for Information Sciences—Permanence of Paper for Printed Library Materials, ANSI Z39.48-1984. ∞ ™

Acquisitions editor: Janet Davis; Project manager: Theresa Rothschadl; Cover designer: Brad Norr; Layout: Cepheus Edmondson

Found an error or a typo? We want to know! Please e-mail it to hapbooks@ache.org, mentioning the book's title and putting "Book Error" in the subject line.

For photocopying and copyright information, please contact Copyright Clearance Center at www.copyright.com or at (978) 750–8400.

Health Administration Press
A division of the Foundation of the American
    College of Healthcare Executives
300 S. Riverside Plaza, Suite 1900
Chicago, IL 60606–6698
(312) 424–2800

For Andrew

Contents

Foreword

Michael H. Covert, FACHE
President and CEO, CHI St. Luke's Health System

ONE MIGHT WONDER why such a successfully published and widely read book (one that has become a must-read for all those entering the profession of healthcare administration) would need to be refreshed. Why would the author add a new emphasis on values—those principles that underlie basic concepts of leadership learned in school, or from mentors, or developed through one's experience in the field?

The answer is quite simple. Our world—our healthcare environment—has evolved to a point that the challenges, opportunities, and stresses we face every day are markedly testing our traditionally held beliefs and values. In fact, we are currently being tested in ways that we never anticipated five or ten years ago.

The personal and work situations that we find ourselves immersed in are causing us to reflect on and evaluate the decisions we make, the people we bring together in team settings to help us make those decisions, and how we best achieve our missions in a matrix environment. Our interactions with others—physicians, employees, boards, vendors, peers, and competitors (who may not have even been trained or employed in the healthcare field)—are causing us to look at ourselves and our profession differently.

This book, now with expanded material, case studies, and questions, gives us the opportunity to pause and assess our status in this new world. What kind of role models have we become or would we like to be for others? How well are we interacting with the team leaders we serve? What have we learned about ourselves, and what can we do to help others grow?

As you read through the chapters, I hope you take time to reflect on your career and your leadership. Think of *Leadership in Healthcare* as a gift from Carson Dye, for it allows you to assess your feelings, beliefs, strengths, and weaknesses in a safe and meaningful way. It also gives you the chance to reinforce and reaffirm those values that are most vital to you. Just as important, it helps you consider changing behaviors, attitudes, and actions to make yourself a better leader—one who is more prepared for the complex future you will face.

Remember, values-based leaders develop teams and individuals who can successfully make structure out of ambiguity. They can handle change and stress during difficult times and learn from those experiences; they recognize the strengths of group interaction and foster environments in which individual contributions are noted and appreciated. They also develop confidence in their ability to effect positive and lasting change in their own organization.

We are in the business of intimacy. Do not let anyone tell you otherwise. It is complicated and demanding *all* of the time. People have entrusted their lives and well-being to you! How do you ensure that this sacred bond is never broken? By constantly testing and reinforcing your values and beliefs to ensure that you stay on the right path.

This third edition of *Leadership in Healthcare* continues to propel you along the self-improvement journey as a true leader in our twenty-first century healthcare field.

Enjoy the read . . .

Academic Foreword

Andrew N. Garman, PsyD
Professor, Rush University, and
CEO, National Center for
Healthcare Leadership

I WRITE THIS foreword during a critical period in the evolution of both healthcare and higher education in the United States. Our country's "eds" and "meds" both deliver critically important services, but both have also grown up on business models that are rapidly outstripping our society's ability to sustain them. While both still enjoy considerable support, we are beginning to recognize that the runaway costs of healthcare and tuition are contributing to levels of economic inequality not seen in this country in more than 80 years.

And yet there is also reason for optimism.

In cities across the country, health systems and universities are recognizing their important status—and responsibilities—as anchor institutions in their local economies. Health systems are recognizing phenomena such as socioeconomic status and income security as social determinants of health and are identifying ways to use both their expertise and purchasing power to foster stronger local economies. Universities are recognizing the importance of ensuring the debt burdens they create for their graduates prove to be sound long-term investments, and they are working with employers to strengthen these returns. Some forward-thinking health systems such as Cleveland Clinic, Northwell, and Kaiser Permanente have begun vertically integrating with university programs to further improve the value proposition for students and employers alike.

But at this time, most of these activities remain outliers. In other cases, they are only experiments: specially funded pilot tests existing tenuously atop a culture of inequity, where long-term health isn't visible above the tyranny of immediate needs. When progress is vulnerable to discretionary budget cuts, the long-term patterns are quick to return.

What will our future look like? Which path will we take? Those questions will be answered by the values we as leaders subscribe to, by how willing we are to take the bold actions needed.

This is where *Leadership in Healthcare* comes in. There are lots of good books out there on the *what* and the *how* of leadership, including *Exceptional Leadership: 16 Critical Competencies for Healthcare Executives*, which Carson and I coauthored. But there are far fewer books on the *why*. *Leadership in Healthcare* was written to address the *why* of leadership. After 17 years and three editions, its longevity is a testament to the importance of its contents.

If you are reading this book as part of a graduate class, you will soon be called upon to lead. If you picked this book up as a practitioner, you may be a leader already. In either case, you probably selected your career path on the basis of deeply held values that you hoped to embody throughout your working life.

I encourage you to read this important book at least twice during your career. On your first read, take special note of the passages that speak to your personal values or articulate things you know in your heart but find difficult to convey to others in words. Bookmark these for later.

Down the road, you will undoubtedly find yourself at your own crossroads in the choices you need to make. These could be times when what you think is right also seems most risky, or times when doing what's best for your community requires considerable sacrifice by the organization that employs you to look after its success. When you find yourself in this space, take out this book again and flip to the pages you bookmarked on your first read. I suspect you will find that reflecting on these passages a second time will help you firm up your convictions while making difficult decisions.

Your values are there for a very important reason: to guide your actions when things get difficult. Now more than ever, we need value-driven leaders.

Like you.

Preface

*Leadership remains a relatively mysterious
concept despite having been studied for several decades.*

—Atul Gupta, Jason C. McDaniel,
and S. Kanthi Herath (2005)

VALUES COME INTO play here.

I wrote *Leadership in Healthcare: Values at the Top*, the first edition of this book, at the turn of the new century. The second edition appeared in 2010. I have been amazed and humbled by its reception. Practitioners and students alike have used it and communicated with me about their reactions, thoughts, and suggestions. I remain humbled by the first edition's selection as the ACHE James Hamilton Book of the Year. I am struck by the power of the message of values in leadership. Yes—values come into play here.

Sixteen years after the publication of the first edition, much has changed in the world, in American society, and in the US healthcare system and its leadership. Yet much remains the same, including the following realities:

1. *Effective leadership is difficult to define.* So many "definitive" leadership books exist, but so few articulate the principles underlying effective leadership.

2. *The ethics of leaders has been on the decline.* Power can corrupt, which is evident from the much-reported unethical and criminal activities of top executives in many industries. When inappropriate conduct is committed in

healthcare, it not only erodes the public's trust but also threatens patients' safety and lives.

3. *The constant stresses in healthcare cause burnout and change of careers.* As a leadership and former search consultant, I am acutely aware of leaders' frustrations and uneasiness about the rapid pace of change in the field. Many of them leave the field as a result, while others struggle through these problems, tired, dejected, and pessimistic.

4. *Leadership development is still not a top priority.* Although many senior executives express an interest in professional growth and development, they devote little time or funds to this pursuit. This paradox is apparent when leadership development becomes the first to get cut from the organizational budget. The economic downturn became another excuse (next to limited time) for overlooking development opportunities.

5. *Effective leaders are almost always values driven.* Those who rely only on hard data and measurable standards often say that values are vague contributors to effectiveness because they cannot be quantified. However, a review of empirical research, coupled with my observations and constant contact with executives, reveals that values are cited by highly effective leaders as major factors of their success.

6. *Effective leadership can be learned.* Some people are "born" leaders. They possess and live by deep, unwavering values. They have a natural ability to interact with and lead others. However, these qualities can be learned by people who are not born with such talents. Becoming aware of the need for learning and practicing a sensitive, practical, and appropriate value system is the first step toward becoming a world-class leader.

In 2010, I wrote, "We now live in a more frenzied, Internet-driven culture, where technology gives to but also takes away from our daily lives." As trite as it may seem, that frenzy has grown, the Internet has more impact than ever before, and technology helps but also hurts us.

I argued then—and I argue even more strongly now—that while technology has allowed us instant access to other people and to enormous amounts of information, it has shrunk our chances for face-to-face communication. The human element is not what it once was. Again, values come into play here.

And while social media—Twitter, Facebook, LinkedIn, and the like—have enabled us to network, stay in touch, and even make "friends" from distant locations, they have also introduced unique challenges in the workplace. Although the Internet age in healthcare has made some veteran executives say that interactions are "not as fun as they used to be," it does attract and excite the younger leaders among us. But once again, values come into play here.

We now live in a world that is very divisive, a country that is polarized, and we work in a healthcare world that has changed enormously. The political, social, and economic uncertainties we face manifest themselves in our healthcare facilities, exacerbating the crises that organizational leaders must solve every day. Emergency departments continue to be the front door and often primary providers of healthcare. We continue to see a shortage in workers, allied health professionals, physicians, and even clinical educators. Retail operators have now entered our world of service and care to others. Financial challenges continue to threaten the availability and quality of care, advances in medical technology and pharmaceuticals have been ramping up the cost of care, and the American public's scrutiny of the healthcare field has gotten closer and deeper. Although not entirely new or insurmountable, these challenges add even more pressure to the already-strained healthcare workforce and its leaders. But once again, values come into play here—and vividly—for our leaders.

Although much progress has been attained in the field, much still needs to be accomplished. This is the environment in which the third edition of *Leadership in Healthcare* is truly effective.

THE INTENT OF THIS BOOK

My goals for this edition are the same as the goals were for the first two editions:

1. Raise leaders' awareness about values and their meaning and applicability to leadership.
2. Posit that values play a major role in leaders' effective performance.
3. Recommend practical strategies for living by those values at work and at home.

Judging by the strong reception to and enduring support for the earlier editions, this book has filled a latent hunger for discussion about values-based leadership, something that even I did not anticipate. The need for such a discussion is not confined to the healthcare executive world; it is also demanded by graduate and undergraduate programs as well as other providers of professional education. The following that the first two editions have garnered has prompted me to present an updated edition that reflects our drastically changed environment.

Changes to the Third Edition

This edition remains true to its original premise. However, to better illustrate and highlight the concepts, I have added new elements and expanded the discussions. These additions further facilitate teaching, dialogue, and self-reflection:

- Chapter 2, "A Review of Academic Leadership Theories and Concepts"
- Chapter 3, "Is the Popular Leadership Literature Worthless?"

- Chapter 21, "The Need for Leaders," written by Christy Harris Lemak, PhD, FACHE
- Chapter 22, "Does Leadership Matter?," written by Patrick D. Shay, PhD
- Appendix D, "Grading Healthcare Team Effectiveness"
- New or expanded treatment of the concepts of servant leadership, change makers, employee engagement, emotional intelligence, and groupthink
- Suggested readings
- New or revised strategies and examples

This edition retains many of the elements of the previous editions:

- Opening vignettes that reflect workplace situations
- Sidebars that support the discussions
- Cases and exercises that stimulate reader response

Content Overview

The book has two forewords—one by Michael H. Covert, FACHE, and another by Andrew N. Garman, PsyD. The rationale here is to represent the perspectives of the book's main audience, which is composed of healthcare executives and health administration educators and students.

The book is divided into five parts. Part I—Leadership in Healthcare—contains chapters 1 through 5 and sets the stage on which the field and its leaders perform their roles. Part II—Personal Values—includes chapters 6 through 12 and catalogs the key values that influence the leader's behaviors, priorities, thought processes, and actions. Part III—Team Values—comprises chapters 13 through 16 and explores the values that guide a leadership team. Part IV—Evaluation—encompasses chapters 17 through 19 and provides guidance for assessing team values and effectiveness and careers at all stages.

The new part V—Academic Perspectives—contains chapters 20 through 22. Chapter 20 is written by Jared D. Lock, PhD, licensed industrial and organizational psychologist and president of The JDL Group LLC. This contribution is a research-based response to and support of the hypotheses offered in the book. Chapter 21 is written by Christy Harris Lemak, PhD, FACHE, professor and chair of the Department of Health Services Administration at the University of Alabama, Birmingham. Her chapter is a well-articulated call for more leadership in healthcare. She is a nationally recognized leader on healthcare administration. Chapter 22 is written by Patrick D. Shay, PhD, assistant professor in the Department of Health Care Administration at Trinity University in San Antonio, Texas. This chapter focuses on academic approaches to the question of whether leadership truly matters in the workplace. Patrick is one of the true up and comers in healthcare administration in organizational behavior and leadership.

Four appendixes are included. Appendixes A through D are tools for evaluating the leader, the team, and the self. The self-evaluation questions in each chapter are designed to challenge current practices and long-held notions about leadership, while all examples (both real and fictional) serve to encourage appropriate behavior and to acknowledge that such model behavior is a multistep, multiyear process that requires willingness, hard work, and other people.

Quotations from various leadership and organizational experts pepper the text throughout, giving credence to the concepts discussed.

CONCLUSION

I have worked in the field for 43 years now, but I continue to learn about and be fascinated by healthcare leadership. I still ask the questions I began posing years ago:

- What is leadership?

- What makes some leaders more effective than others?
- What role do values play in leadership?
- How can people improve their own leadership skills?

Although this book is not a complete treatise on leadership, it does explore concepts that will cause you to reflect on your own and others' value systems, behaviors, leadership competencies, mindsets, actions, goals, and performance. I hope it communicates these messages:

1. Values come into play in leadership.
2. Effective leadership is needed now more than ever.
3. Values-based leadership can be learned.
4. Values are a primary contributor to great leadership performance.

I share what several individuals have said about values:

Tell me what you pay attention to, and I will tell you who you are.
—*José Ortega y Gasset (1958)*

Values-based leadership may not be a cure for everything that ails us, but it's definitely a good place to start.
—*Harry M. Jansen Kraemer Jr. (2011)*

Sometimes it takes great moral courage to do what is right, even when the right action seems clear.
—*Richard L. Hughes, Robert C. Ginnett, and Gordon J. Curphy (2015)*

In today's world, the amount of distraction and busyness we all experience keeps us from undertaking the inward journey and engaging in the quiet reflection required to become more authentic human beings.

—*Kevin Cashman (2008)*

Leaders need to understand explicitly what they stand for, because values provide a prism through which all behavior is ultimately viewed.

—*James M. Kouzes and Barry Z. Posner (2012)*

The rest, as Lao Tzu said, is up to you.

Carson F. Dye, FACHE

REFERENCES

Cashman, K. 2008. *Leadership from the Inside Out: Becoming a Leader for Life*, 2nd ed. San Francisco: Berrett-Kohler Publishers, Inc.

Gupta, A., J. C. McDaniel, and S. K. Herath. 2005. "Quality Management in Service Firms: Sustaining Structures of Total Quality Service." *Managing Service Quality* 15 (4): 389–402.

Hughes, R. L., R. C. Ginnett, and G. J. Curphy. 2015. *Leadership: Enhancing the Lessons of Experience*, 8th ed. Burr Ridge, IL: McGraw-Hill Education.

Kouzes, J. M., and B. Z. Posner. 2012. *The Leadership Challenge: How to Make Extraordinary Things Happen in Organizations*, 5th ed. San Francisco: Jossey-Bass.

Kraemer, H. M. J. Jr. 2011. "The Only True Leadership Is Values-Based Leadership." Published April 26. www.forbes.com/2011/04/26/values-based-leadership.html.

Ortega y Gasset, J. 1958. *Man and Crisis*. Translated by Mildred Adams. New York: W. W. Norton & Co.

INSTRUCTOR RESOURCES

This book's Instructor Resources include PowerPoint slides for each chapter, additional discussion questions, and web links.

For the most up-to-date information about this book and its Instructor Resources, go to ache.org/HAP and browse for the book's title or author name.

This book's Instructor Resources are available to instructors who adopt this book for use in their course. For access information, please e-mail hapbooks@ache.org.

Acknowledgments

I HAVE WORKED—no, lived, really lived—in healthcare for more than 40 years. (They say once you move past 40 years, you shouldn't be quite so precise.) My entire career has been marked by interaction with leaders. From Sister Mary George, RSM, first CEO of Clermont Mercy Hospital, and my first boss in healthcare, to the wide-ranging group of leaders participating in my last ACHE workshop, my career has focused on identifying strong leaders, coaching and counseling leaders at all levels, guiding physicians as they begin their own leadership journeys, and serving clients in hundreds of executive searches. All of these thousands of individuals should be acknowledged—but alas, they are too numerous to be listed.

My good fortune has been compounded by working for and with some exemplary leaders. While that list would also be too lengthy to include in this preface, I do think of Sister Mary George, Michael Covert, Donald Cramp, and the late Dr. Lonnie Wright and Sy Sokatch from Children's Hospital in Cincinnati. Michael Covert was a great leader to work for and was also gracious enough to once again write the practitioner foreword for this third edition. Other leaders have given me the chance to recruit them, recruit for them, counsel them, help them on board, and work with their boards and senior teams. All of these leaders have had a significant influence on my thinking: Dr. Scott Ransom, Dr. Lee Hammerling, Randy Oostra, Dr. Mark Peters, Michael Ugwueke, Kevin Spiegel, Chip Hubbs, Kris Hoce, Dr. Scot Remick, Dr. Kathleen Forbes, Tim Putnam, Larry Gumina, Scott Malaney, Bill Linesch, Dr. Greg

Taylor, Dr. Akram Boutros, Jack Janoso, Bruce Hagen, Dr. John Byrnes, Dr. David James, Dr. John Paris, and Dr. Bob Kiskaddon. Moreover, having the ability to work alongside Kam Sigafoos, Bill Sanger, Gene Miyamoto, the late Dr. Ed Pike, Mike Gilligan, Mark Hannahan, Mark Elliott, Walter McLarty, Gretchen Patton, and Randy Schimmoeller gave me great day-to-day lessons in leadership.

It's all about values, and these individuals represent great values. I have watched them and learned much from them. Often, they were unaware that I was making mental notes on what they did and how effective they were in their leadership activities. But their behavior always came back to their inherent values. These are the leaders of our healthcare enterprises in America, and because of their values, we can stand confidently knowing our healthcare organizations are in their hands.

Over the years it has been an honor and a privilege to teach in the academy. My academic career began at the University of Cincinnati in the summer of 1977, continued with Xavier University from 1978 to 1981, and grew with Dr. Steve Strasser at the Ohio State University from 1985 to 2007. I have been honored to teach at the University of Alabama, Birmingham, for the past seven years. All this classroom time has given me the impetus to grow in my academic knowledge of leadership. I find myself always going to the scholarly articles section of Google before reading the popular literature. My hope is that more practitioners will turn to the evidence-based literature, and more frequently.

Appreciation also goes to the various faculty who have chosen this book for their leadership courses. I am honored that I can be of some assistance as they fulfill the calling of preparing tomorrow's healthcare leaders. Thank you all.

While waxing scholarly, I would like to acknowledge Andrew Garman, my friend, colleague, and occasional coauthor. Andy brings a true scholarly focus to his work and outlook, and I have benefited from my work with him. He was kind enough to provide the academic foreword for this book, and I am in his debt.

The second edition of this book was written in 2010, during a time of great upheaval in healthcare. Yet today's changes are proving to be much more turbulent. My counsel as a leadership consultant, my work as an executive search consultant, and my focus on leadership assessment give me exposure to exceptional leaders every day. These individuals practice values-based leadership, and I always gain from my exposure to them. Each and every day is an exciting day of learning for me. I am so fortunate to have had this career.

Finally, conducting workshops, training sessions, and webinars for healthcare associations and other organizations continues to expand my understanding of leadership concepts.

Health Administration Press (HAP) is *our* publisher for our industry. We are quite lucky to have them. They dedicate their hours and days to finding authors who can expand our understanding and help us do more effective work and service. Their publications are timely and high in quality. I want to acknowledge and praise them. Specifically, I am grateful for the leadership of Michael Cunningham and Janet Davis. Janet pushed me to do this third edition, and she was right—her suggestions have made this a much more powerful leadership text. She has always been a great supporter and friend, and I truly value that. My editor, Theresa Rothschadl, was tireless and always optimistic. Until you have the chance to work with an editor at this level, you cannot know the closeness that grows. Your editor seems to be present at every meal and every thought. Lest you think this was agonizing, I must say that Theresa made the process easy. She is incredibly thorough, humorous (yes, humorous), adept at editing an academic book, and remarkably interactive. She has deep feelings for her thoughts and suggestions, and her input made this book far better. Thanks, Theresa!

Big thanks to Jared Lock, Christy Lemak, and Patrick Shay. These three distinguished healthcare leaders and academics provided expert authority on academic aspects of leadership. Their contributions have made this book far stronger. I cherish their three offerings.

I said this in the second edition and I repeat it here: To work and serve in such a distinctive field as healthcare is a calling and a blessing. Healthcare has so many devoted, values-driven leaders who deserve much credit and acknowledgment. Again, I also acknowledge those many men and women in uniform with whom I work so often—the Army, Air Force, Navy Medical Service Corps, Medical Corps, and Nursing Corps. Many of them gave me great leadership lessons, including David Rubenstein, Paul Williamson, Kathy Van Der Linden, Steve Wooldridge, Kyle Campbell, Patrick Misnick, and Mark Wilhite. I salute and thank them.

My most important acknowledgment always goes to my family. They have missed me often as I traveled the country working with leaders, and yet they are always my greatest sources of support and love. So I acknowledge my four wonderful daughters, Carly, Emily, Liesl, and Blakely; a great son-in-law, Jeremy; three grandsons, Carson, Benjamin, and Andrew; and Philippe Larouche. As usual, Liesl helped with some editing input and graphic counsel. My wife, Joaquina, has always supported my writing and has often made it much more logical.

This book has been a very special one for me. I was greatly honored with its selection in 2001 as the ACHE James A. Hamilton Book of the Year. While this third edition marks my eleventh book, *Leadership in Healthcare* maintains its unique position. The book represents my belief in values-driven leadership and how each of us carries part of those with whom we work and interact into our own leadership styles. In the musical *Wicked,* the story of the witches in *The Wizard of Oz,* these words are shared between Glinda, the "good" witch, and Elphaba, the "bad" witch:

> I've heard it said
> That people come into our lives for a reason
> Bringing something we must learn
> And we are led
> To those who help us most to grow
> If we let them
> And we help them in return

Well, I don't know if I believe that's true
But I know I'm who I am today
Because I knew you.

Thanks to you leaders out there—because I knew you, I have greatly grown in my understanding of leadership.

Carson F. Dye, FACHE

PART I

LEADERSHIP IN HEALTHCARE

CHAPTER 1

The Leadership Imperative

We are crossing a line into a territory with
unpredictable turmoil and exponentially growing
change—change for which we are not prepared.

—John Kotter (2014)

UNIVERSITY MEDICAL CENTER is hosting an annual reception for its retired employees. Jonathan Sneed, the medical center's CEO in the 1980s, is one of the special guests. Now in his 80s, Jonathan remains sharp as he sits at a table with Elizabeth Jankowski, the current CEO. The two are discussing the evolution of healthcare management.

JONATHAN. Elizabeth, your challenges are more complex than ours were 40 years ago. Back then, we thought our issues were insurmountable! But I suspect that 25 years from now, you'll think your problems now are simple. There's one constant necessity for a leader throughout the years, however. Leaders have to be constantly learning and adjusting their skills and knowledge. They always have to anticipate what's coming just past the horizon. This leadership quality has kept this academic medical center at the forefront and contributed to its great reputation as a learning organization.

ELIZABETH. Great point! I do get concerned sometimes about some of our leaders. In fact, last week at our senior council meeting, we talked about how so many of us have become so busy that we haven't been able to invest time in leadership education. There are days we just put out fires. The constant e-mails and interruptions from our so-called smartphones rule more and more of our time. We just don't have the chance to do the strategic deep dive that I know we need.

JONATHAN. Watch out for that. Not keeping up with the trends and the new realities is like not changing the oil in your car often enough. You won't see the negative effects until it's too late.

"IT WAS THE best of times, it was the worst of times," writes Charles Dickens in his classic book *A Tale of Two Cities.* The same can be said of constantly evolving healthcare. Consider some of the realities (both good and bad) in the field that confront healthcare leaders today:

- Shift from volume to value
- Clinical integration
- Transparency
- Population health management
- Management of the continuum of care—and care moving out of the acute care setting
- Consolidation, alliances, affiliations, and consortiums among providers
- Professional shortages and decreasing recruitment pools
- Retail incursion into healthcare
- Continuing pressures of Big Data—more and more issues with electronic health record systems and other clinical and information technologies

- Impact of the Internet
- Patient use of smartphones
- Aging population
- Changes in worker and patient ethnic and cultural demographics
- Higher expectations from consumers; consumerism
- Loss of public respect for the healthcare field

These challenges, and those yet to come, are exactly why the leadership imperative exists. The leadership imperative is the need for healthcare executives to enhance their understanding of the forces at play in the field and the way they manage through these changes. Leaders must now build judicious forecasts by thinking in the long term and changing these forecasts more frequently than every three years (the current traditional strategic plan cycle). The imperative demands planning that goes past the current workday or budget year. Simply put, the healthcare field, its workers, and the people it serves need leaders who can rebuild trust; restore efficient processes; and ensure quality through uncertain environmental trends and practices, societal and economic flux, and organizational transitions.

EVOLVING ENVIRONMENT

Healthcare's evolution has brought not just improvements. In fact, it has created inefficiencies and disorganization. However, it has also ushered in more jobs, better operating standards and clinical outcomes, lifesaving advances, a focus on patients and disease management, improved services, and new sources of revenue (among other things).

Current trends (listed in exhibit 1.1) and common obstacles (discussed later in the chapter) shape the healthcare environment in which workers function and services are provided. In this landscape, physician–organization relations continue to be among the most challenging

Exhibit 1.1 Current Trends in Healthcare

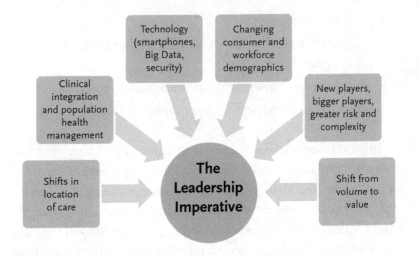

issues, along with strategic conflicts that could result from mergers or other steps to gain economies of scale or increase market share. Such conflicts may derail the flow of decisions and disrupt patient services.

Amid changes and problems, healthcare leaders plow through. Some are weary and doubtful of their ability to rebuild trust and continue to guide their organizations. Some, however, are energized by the challenges. When I have asked about the current state of the field, several healthcare executives make the following comments:

- "These are very tough times to be leading a hospital, but I would not have it any other way. This is a good test of my leadership."
- "Well, when the going gets tough, the tough get going— that is certainly true today. I am really up for the challenge."
- "After 35 years in this field, I thought I had seen it all, but the changes keep coming. I am OK with that, but it certainly gets tiring many days."

- "I have a better view and sense of direction here at the top. But I am concerned about my middle managers who are down in the trenches. I need to do whatever I can to help them keep holding on."

As these responses articulate, this era is both an exhausting and an exciting time to be a leader in healthcare.

COMMON OBSTACLES AND IMPERATIVE ACTIONS

Aside from coping with the current realities of the field, healthcare leaders also navigate the common obstacles of running multifaceted operations. In this section, these obstacles are listed along with an appropriate imperative action. An imperative action is a step that a leader may take to overcome the obstacle.

Obstacle 1: Organizations Today Are More Complex

Until the 1990s, healthcare organizations were structured in a relatively simple manner. Free-standing hospitals, private doctor's offices, nursing homes, and local pharmacies were the most ubiquitous embodiments of organizations. Healthcare *systems* did not exist, nor did integrated delivery networks and nursing home chains, and few mergers and acquisitions took place. Physicians were not employed by health systems; instead, they ran small, independent practices.

A hospital was not a conglomerate; it existed solely to provide care for the hospitalized patient. Therefore, its leaders were not mired in the politics

> The problems of making healthcare work are large. The complexities are overwhelming governments, economies, and societies around the world. We have every indication, however, that where people in medicine combine their talents and efforts to design organized service to patients and local communities, extraordinary change can result.
>
> —Atul Gawande (2011)

of multiple business partners or the bureaucracy of multiple service lines. A hospital's mission and vision were clear.

"The more complex the system, the less efficient its operation" is an adage that is true of today's healthcare systems. Decreased efficiency results in less satisfaction not only for the system's patients but also for its workers. Complex systems exhaust leaders and resources because they require more attention and focus.

Imperative action: Restore the simplicity of the healthcare organization by clarifying its structure, mission and vision, and future direction. Work to minimize the complexities of intricate organizational structures.

Obstacle 2: Employee Engagement and Loyalty Are Low

Opinion surveys continue to reveal that employee commitment and engagement are decreasing. According to Gallup (2016), "A staggering 87% of employees worldwide are not engaged at work. The world has a crisis of engagement—one with serious and potentially long-lasting repercussions for the global economy."

Job security is one of the most important elements of a high-performance work environment. For a long time, healthcare offered just that: job security. Employees, in turn, showed their appreciation for this security by being loyal to the organization. Employees stayed at their jobs longer, performed harder and better, recommended family members and friends to apply for open positions, missed fewer workdays, and participated more in the activities of the organization. Gallup has developed a well-known employee engagement tool and has shown that engaged employees are more productive (Adkins 2016).

Today, even the hardiest healthcare systems cannot ensure jobs for their employees. One CEO suggests that the high levels of trust between management and staff that once existed in the healthcare field may never return: "I remember the first time I faced a room full of hospital employees who were to be laid off. That was 15 years ago, and I personally talked to all of them. However, the last three times my organization has laid employees off, I did not even go to the sessions. I was told that it was legally risky and that it could be better handled by our human resources staff. We handed the laid-off employees to an outplacement firm. I feel like I abandoned them and feel really bad, but I don't know what to do about it."

> **Imperative action:** Enlist the engagement of strong employees by boosting trust levels and encouraging their participation in organizational initiatives, such as by giving them increased personal control and decision-making roles.

Obstacle 3: Physicians Are Increasingly Disengaged and Dissatisfied with the Field

Physicians aged 55 or older have different expectations from those who are just beginning medical practice. Older physicians have witnessed the growth of managed care and eventual drops in reimbursement. They have experienced financial and legal challenges to their role as the "captain of the ship" in patient care. They mourn the disappearance of the club-like atmosphere of medicine, filled with people with the same concerns and priorities. The transition to electronic health records has tried the patience of many. Some physicians even regret having entered the profession.

Younger physicians, on the other hand, have different expectations. Most, if not all, of them begin their careers with enormous student loan debts (some estimates suggest $170,000 or more—see Association of American Medical Colleges 2014), so they desire stable employment with set hours and salary. In addition, younger physicians believe that medicine is only one part of their life, while older physicians put most of their lives' focus on medicine. These divergent perspectives and work styles have caused tension between these two groups.

> The world is now changing at a rate at which the basic systems, structures, and cultures built over the past century cannot keep up with the demands being placed on them. Incremental adjustments to how you manage and strategize, no matter how clever, are not up to the job.
>
> —John Kotter (2014)

The practice of employing physicians, which was the trend in the 1990s, has returned. While in the 1990s hospitals and health systems hired doctors in response to capitated care financing, today the reason is a combination of physicians' pursuit of a more secure employment (as opposed to the difficulty and expense of private practice and the high rates for malpractice insurance) and the organizations' need for physician loyalty (Accenture 2015). Although physician employment can help align common interests and goals, it may also reduce the physicians' autonomy and complicate their decision making. As a result, physicians, even employed ones, may end up losing faith in and loyalty to the organization. If given a choice, many physicians would rather have another physician as the leader of the organization, as this actual sentiment from a hospital physician board member underscores: "We seem to have forgotten our patients in our drive to build a bigger, more comprehensive healthcare system. At least having a physician as our CEO would bring back that patient focus."

The many significant changes within the field are enticing many physicians to move into leadership. Bisordi and Aboujoud (2015) report that "from payors and providers to facilities such as hospitals where services are delivered, healthcare reform has ushered in an era where physician leadership is, quite simply, essential for long-term success." Graduate schools throughout the country have developed management programs targeted at physicians. Multiple healthcare organizations have created physician leadership development academies. Many physicians enrolled in these courses are motivated by their dissatisfaction with how healthcare organizations are managed. These doctors seek to improve these facilities' operations and services as well as gain more influence over the strategic directions of their organizations.

Imperative action: Improve relations with the physician collective. Handle physician employment skillfully. Consider the fact that more and more physicians are needed in leadership roles. Build robust physician leadership development programs. Make room for the increasing number of part-time physician leaders who will remain in some clinical practice.

Obstacle 4: Pay for Value and Clinical Integration

Perhaps there is no greater change to the healthcare field than the radical shift in payment methods brought about by the Affordable Care Act of 2010. Healthcare provision had been built on the concept of volume. It was a very simple-to-understand business in one respect: Bring more patients in the door, get paid for it, and business was good. "More heads in beds" was the mantra. While talking about the so-called shift to a value-based reimbursement scheme is easy, guiding a real institution through the enormous changes it brought about—managing across that chasm—is almost frightening in its complexity. Feyman (2014) states, "Despite some shining examples of success, value-based payments have a nastier side as well." In fact, evidence suggests that there are no savings at all in some programs.

Clinical integration will create benefits for patients but massive changes for the field. Improvements include "the elimination of duplicate clinical and administrative work, a common patient record that ensures that the status of the patient is tracked throughout the entire course of care with no continuity-of-care gaps, a reduced chance of errors, systematic support of best practices and evidence-based care, and full alignment of the goals of all providers" (Dye and Sokolov 2013, 104). But as Faber (2016) states, "Some systems that have invested in clinical integration will go out of business or be acquired by more successful systems, which in turn will downsize or divest those facilities."

Imperative action: Carefully craft logical strategic and tactical initiatives to shift toward value-based reimbursement and clinical integration without harming the care enterprise.

Obstacle 5: Patients Are Dissatisfied with Healthcare

Staggering healthcare costs, high insurance premiums or narrow-network insurance plans, poor quality of care, limited access to care, and lack of attention or information from providers are just some concerns that cause patient dissatisfaction. A survey by Prophet and GE Healthcare Camden Group (2016) shows that "81 percent of consumers are dissatisfied with their health care experience." The same study showed a 3 percent decline in patient satisfaction from 2013 to 2014.

Moreover, despite calls for improvement, quality and patient safety remain a serious challenge in the United States. According to McCann (2014), "Preventable medical errors persist as the No. 3 killer in the U.S.—third only to heart disease and cancer—claiming the lives of some 400,000 people each year" (see also James 2013). Many patient safety advocates, including the Institute for Healthcare Improvement, have raised the level of awareness about dissatisfaction and have pushed various quality practices. The field has made some progress in this regard, but unfortunately, quality is just one of the many areas that need to be addressed.

Many healthcare systems have grown so large that patients report a lack of responsiveness similar to that experienced with large corporations. One educated patient compares her experiences with her health system to "calling an 800 customer service number in the middle of the night on Sunday." In a consumer-driven healthcare market, this type of treatment could lead to loss of revenue, at best, and loss of patient trust, at worst.

> **Imperative action:** Make quality of care and patient safety your number-one priority. Pay attention to consumer service, and establish good relationships with the communities you serve.

Obstacle 6: Succession Planning Is Not a Priority for Some Retiring Leaders

An increasing number of baby boomer executives will retire in the next few years. Despite these retirement plans, many leaders have not developed succession plans to ensure that their transitions are handled effectively.

Next-generation leaders are ready and waiting for their opportunity to learn and grow in these management roles. Many are aware of the leadership imperative and are confident and excited about the future, although some are fearful of current trends.

Imperative action: Invest time and resources in succession planning and leadership development programs to ensure that the new generation of leaders will make the significant inroads and positive contributions needed for high-quality patient care and service to their communities.

CONCLUSION

The title of this chapter, "The Leadership Imperative," stems from two of the most urgent issues in healthcare today. First, leadership in healthcare is undeniably important, so the field needs a leadership book solely dedicated to healthcare. Healthcare is, in fact, different from other fields. As Gawande (2014, 6) writes, "Scientific advances have turned the process of aging and dying into medical experiments, matters to be managed by health care professionals. And we in the medical world have proved alarmingly unprepared for it." Leadership must walk side by side with healers and help remove barriers to success. Second, massive changes are transpiring in healthcare. Again, Gawande (2011) says it best: "You are the generation on the precipice of a transformation medicine has no choice but to undergo, the riders in the front car of the roller coaster clack-clack-clacking its way up to the drop. The revolution that remade how other fields handle complexity is coming to health care, and I think you sense it." Heeding the leadership imperative and taking up this mantle is what is required of leaders in healthcare today. Are you ready and willing?

But while the challenges facing healthcare are exceptional, some problems of leadership are classic. Root, a firm that helps organizations bridge the gaps in strategy and foster employees' understanding of that strategy and willingness to engage in it, presents a very unusual visual called *The Canyon* (see exhibit 1.2). Jim Haudan (2016), CEO of Root, describes it: "*The Canyon* reflects the reality of people's day-to-day jobs at all levels and functions of an organization. Dealing with those realities is the first step toward creating engaged employees and executing strategies like superstars. When leaders don't face reality head-on, it does not bode well for goal achievement."

Haudan (2016) further explains:

> What the image really shows are these canyons between the leaders of an organization who can see what needs to be done but don't have their hands on the levers of change every day, the managers stuck somewhere between the leaders and the doers so that they must balance a lack of full information with a need for employee guidance, and the doers who have their hands on change every day but can't see what needs to be done. So what you find, and maybe even metaphorically, is that everybody is at a different altitude, and everybody sees the problems that we face very differently.
>
> You know we have this wonderful saying: "People will tolerate the conclusions of their leaders, but they will act on their own." But if you are going to change the dynamic of that, which means that everybody is in a different corner, and that our conclusions are similar, then what we see in terms of our businesses must be explored equally. So everybody—leaders, managers, and individuals—must be able to see all the drama in the business and given the decency to compare and contrast, to check and recheck, to unlearn and to relearn, and when they are given that opportunity 99.9 percent of people come to very similar conclusions.
>
> The problem is what each of us sees is so different, our conclusions are so different, that again these canyons get perpetuated.

Building bridges across the Canyon is, I think, the leadership imperative.

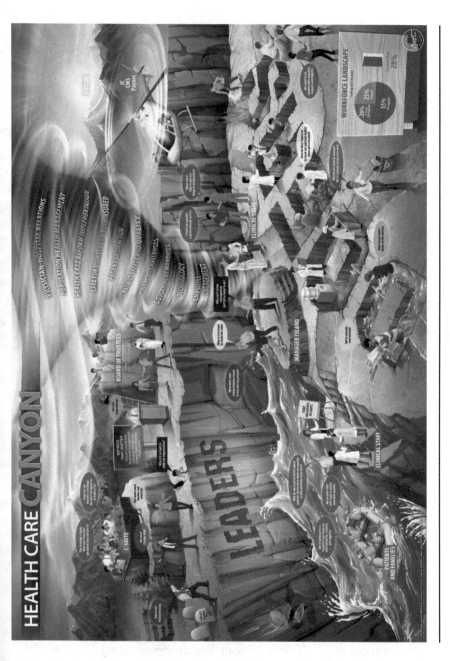

Source: The Canyon® is reprinted with permission. This Strategic Learning Map® visual is a product of Root Inc., Sylvania, OH 43560, www.rootinc.com ©2015.

Self-Evaluation Questions

❑ Do I view myself as a leader? If so, is my goal to bring about needed change or, in the words of one CEO, "to build palaces and monuments to my legacy"?

❑ Do I view leadership as an act, a process, or a skill?

❑ Do I, and other leaders I know, think that a leadership imperative exists today?

❑ Have I observed any significant shifts and trends in the field and popular culture that affect leadership in my organization?

❑ Does it seem more difficult to lead and manage change today?

❑ What does the illustration of the Canyon mean to you as a leader?

Exercise
Exercise 1.1
Read and reflect on the following article. Outline the primary areas of concern for healthcare leaders, and suggest steps that could reduce the problems created by generation gaps.

Lim, A., and T. Epperly. 2013. "Generation Gap: Effectively Leading Physicians of All Ages." *Family Practice Management* 20 (3): 29–34.

REFERENCES

Accenture. 2015. "Clinical Care: The (Independent) Doctor Will NOT See You Now." Accessed April 1, 2016. www.accenture.

com/_acnmedia/PDF-2/Accenture-The-Doctor-Will-Not-See-You.pdf.

Adkins, A. 2016. "Employee Engagement in U.S. Stagnant in 2015." Gallup. Published January 13. www.gallup.com/poll/188144/employee-engagement-stagnant-2015.aspx.

Association of American Medical Colleges. 2014. *Medical Student Education: Debt, Costs, and Loan Repayment Fact Card.* Published October. https://members.aamc.org/eweb/upload/2014%20DFC_%20vertical.pdf.

Bisordi, J., and M. Abouljoud. 2015. "Physician Leadership Initiatives at Small or Mid-size Organizations." *Healthcare.* Published October 20. http://dx.doi.org/10.1016/j.hjdsi.2015.08.008.

Dye, C. F., and J. J. Sokolov. 2013. *Developing Physician Leaders for Successful Clinical Integration.* Chicago: Health Administration Press.

Faber, W. 2016. "Clinical Integration: There Will Be Winners and Losers." LinkedIn. Published February 11. www.linkedin.com/pulse/clinical-integration-winners-losers-william-faber.

Feyman, Y. 2014. "Where Is the Value in Health Care?" *Forbes.* Published July 21. www.forbes.com/sites/theapothecary/2014/07/21/where-is-the-value-in-health-care/#7884657f66b0.

Gallup. 2016. "The Culture of an Engaged Workplace: Q12 Engagement." Accessed March 30. www.gallup.com/services/169328/q12-employee-engagement.aspx.

Gawande, A. 2014. *Being Mortal.* New York: Metropolitan Books.

———. 2011. "Cowboys and Pit Crews." *New Yorker.* Published May 26. www.newyorker.com/news/news-desk/cowboys-and-pit-crews.

Haudan, J. 2016. Interview with author, April 3.

James, J. T. 2013. "A New, Evidence-Based Estimate of Patient Harms Associated with Hospital Care." *Journal of Patient Safety* 9 (3): 122–28.

Kotter, J. 2014. *Accelerate: Building Strategic Agility for a Faster-Moving World.* Boston: Harvard Business Review Press.

McCann, E. 2014. "Deaths by Medical Mistakes Hit Records." *Healthcare IT News.* Published July 18. www.healthcareit news.com/news/deaths-by-medical-mistakes-hit-records.

Prophet and GE Healthcare Camden Group. 2016. *The State of Consumer Healthcare: A Study of Patient Experience.* Accessed April 1. www.prophet.com/patientexperience/.

SUGGESTED READINGS

Haeder, S. F., and D. L. Weimer. 2013. "You Can't Make Me Do It: State Implementation of Insurance Exchanges Under the Affordable Care Act." In "The Health Care Crucible Post-Reform: Challenges for Public Administration," edited by Frank J. Thompson. Special issue. *Public Administration Review* 73 (1): S34–S47.

Jha, A. K., K. E. Joynt, J. Orav, and A. M. Epstein. 2012. "The Long-Term Effect of Premier Pay for Performance on Patient Outcomes." *New England Journal of Medicine* 366 (17): 1606–15.

Keckley, P. 2016. "Is Healthcare Ripe for Disintermediation?" *Pulse Weekly.* Navigant Consulting. Published January 19. www. naviganthrp.com/is-healthcare-ripe-for-disintermediation/.

Kocher, R., and N. R. Sahni. 2011. "Hospitals' Race to Employ Physicians—The Logic Behind a Money-Losing Proposition." *New England Journal of Medicine* 364 (19): 1790–93.

McDonough, J. E. 2012. "The Road Ahead for the Affordable Care Act." *New England Journal of Medicine* 367(3): 199–201.

Rosenthal, M. B. 2008. "Beyond Pay for Performance—Emerging Models of Provider-Payment Reform." *New England Journal of Medicine* 359 (12): 1197–200.

Swenson, S. J., G. S. Meyer, E. C. Nelson, G. C. Hunt, D. B. Pryor, J. I. Weissberg, G. S. Kaplan, J. Daley, G. R. Yates, M. R. Chassin, B. C. James, and D. M. Berwick. 2010. "Cottage Industry to Postindustrial Care—The Revolution in Health Care Delivery." *New England Journal of Medicine* 362 (5): e12.

A Review of Academic Leadership Theories and Concepts

Leadership is a complex and diverse topic, and trying to make sense of leadership research can be an intimidating endeavor.

—David V. Day and John Antonakis (2012)

DR. MALCOLM LEARNED of Somewhere State University opened a health administration lecture with the question, "What is leadership?" Students offered the following responses:

- Getting groups of people to follow you.
- Using power appropriately to meet organizational objectives.
- The process of uniting individuals into groups to serve a vision or a mission.
- In the past, leadership was all about power, but today it's about influence.
- Understanding the global purpose of an organization and giving direction to subordinates to ensure their work is serving that purpose.
- It is engagement.
- It stands for the position and the activity of making change and moving toward a goal.

- Leadership comes down to having interpersonal skills, and it really is something that you are born with. Some people are just leaders, and others are just followers.
- Using a set of skills to make improvements in society or in organizations.
- Getting results. In instances when the leader abuses his or her power, the results may not be good. But in other cases, the results are beneficial to all those concerned.
- Although it may not be politically correct to say, leadership is all about power. This power can be used to coerce people into doing things they would not do otherwise.

Dr. Learned closed the discussion by asking, "Did you hear how disparate the answers to my question were? If we all have different definitions, how can we study leadership, and how can we improve ourselves as leaders?"

Guide to the Reader
Academic theories of leadership, though they sometimes seem opaque and confusing, can provide a great foundation for better understanding how to enhance one's leadership skills and competencies. Each theory has some piece of wisdom and some grain of significant truth.

LEADERSHIP IS ONE of the most discussed and, ultimately, the most misunderstood concepts in management. Is it an art, a science, or both? Is leadership defined by the act, the process, or the skill? Is a person a leader because she is in charge of moving a team from Point A to Point B? Is someone a leader because he has followers? What is the mark of a good leader, and does it matter how a leader achieves greatness? Are leaders born or are they made? Or both?

As a long-time leadership consultant, teacher, and executive recruiter, I have noticed that "you know what I mean" is one of the most repeated phrases during my discussions with employers about what qualities they are looking for in a leader. Although employers offer their favorite general descriptors of a qualified leader—for example, "an outstanding communicator" who has "integrity and high energy" and is "a people person, a team player, and results oriented"—they are hard-pressed to provide specific details of what they mean. As a result, these employers resort to replying with the statement, "Well, you know what I mean—I just want a strong leader." After all the publications, seminars, speeches, and casual banter about leadership, few leaders can actually articulate a comprehensive definition of leadership.

Leadership is a living phenomenon; therefore, it is expected to change shape according to its purpose and the demands of its followers and the environment. This adaptability is probably why a definition is so elusive.

The first two editions of this book provided a brief review of the academic theories of leadership. To provide a more comprehensive review, this new edition delves into the rich academic history of leadership theory. Doing so is pertinent for three reasons. First, because the book is used significantly in health administration programs (graduate and undergraduate), a more inclusive examination will enhance students' understanding of leadership as they prepare to enter leadership roles in healthcare. Second, the study of leadership in higher education has grown substantively over the past several years. Many colleges and universities now offer majors in leadership. Third, and perhaps most important, looking first to research-based studies is vital to better understanding what leadership is and how it is practiced. While there is likely some art to leadership, there is also science. That science should be studied and understood.

Currently, many books and articles on leadership are, in fact, *not* based on any credible evidence. Instead, they contain anecdotal observations and are based only on the subjective and often one-sided notions of the authors. This problem will become more apparent to the reader after finishing chapter 3, which examines popular leadership literature—comprising many books that, frankly, are not supported by evidence.

CHRONOLOGICAL REVIEW OF LEADERSHIP

One common way to study academic leadership theories is through a chronological historical review. Although the concept of leadership has probably been around since prehistoric days, the discussion in this chapter begins in the late 1800s. As the changes brought about by the Industrial Revolution became a more significant part of society, the German sociologist Max Weber wrote about bureaucracy and the benefits of organizing people into groups. He focused on the use of structure and power, viewing people largely as cogs in the overall production machine. Management theorists Henri Fayol and Frederick Taylor examined span of control and scientific management, respectively. While neither Fayol nor Taylor was an academic or thinking of the topic of leadership, their thoughts have long-term impact on the study of leadership.

Great Man Theory (1900 Through the 1940s)

As the Industrial Revolution gained full force, attention began to focus on how leaders (often called *managers* at this time) were identified. Essentially, the question facing the owners of factories was, "How can I pinpoint the person in the workforce who has the best ability to control the others?" The first major group of theories assumed that the best leaders were born that way and were thus "great men." Note that a feature of the great man theory continues to have great popular support (as opposed to evidence-based validation) because many individuals today believe that strong leaders possess charisma, intelligence, or inborn talent that makes them effective. However, evidence did not support this view for long—not all great leaders are men, and not all individuals with the identified inborn characteristics become great leaders. Leadership was shown to be more complex, and success hinged on many other factors.

Trait Theory (1920s Through the Present)

The great man theory morphed into the study and categorization of the characteristics of leaders and became known as trait theory. The two world wars provided impetus to this study. Faced with a critical challenge of determining who should be officers and lead other soldiers, sailors, and airmen, the US armed forces decided that if they could simply come up with a list of the qualities, attributes, or talents inherent in leaders, they could make effective decisions in selecting officers. Trait theory essentially attempts to identity those personality factors, characteristics, or qualities that effective leaders possess. Some examples include confidence, high energy, initiative, drive, decision-making ability, and creativity. A more recent example is emotional intelligence.

Great man theory and trait theory, although not well supported by long-term research findings, still form the foundation of many contemporary popular views of leadership. Many participants in leadership workshops answer the question, "What is a leader?" with descriptions related to traits or inborn characteristics. Exhibit 2.1 provides a visual picture of both theories and their common critiques.

Contingency and Situational Leadership Theories (1940s Through the Present)

In the 1930s and 1940s, interest in the academic study of leadership began in earnest. Perhaps the harbinger of this was Chester Barnard, author of the well-known *The Functions of the Executive* (1938). Although not an academic but rather an executive at AT&T and later chair of the National Science Foundation, Barnard (1938, 87) wrote that leadership was the "ability of a superior to influence the behavior of a subordinate or group and persuade them to follow a particular course of action." In contrast to earlier leadership theories, Gabor and Mahoney (2013, 136) note that Barnard "viewed the organization as a complex social system."

Exhibit 2.1 Early Leadership Theories: Great Man Theory and Trait Theory

GREAT MAN THEORY	TRAIT THEORY

CENTRAL IDEAS

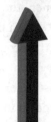

- Heredity plays a significant role in who is a leader.
- Leaders are born, not made.

- Intelligence, personal drive, and extraversion are inborn and mark great leaders.
- Knowing the traits of effective leaders makes it easier to identify them.

CRITIQUES

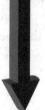

- Leadership skills can be developed through proper education and experience.
- No scientific evidence exists showing why leaders become effective.

- No exclusive set of traits is appropriate across differing situations.
- Theory is inward-looking and ignores followers and situational tasks.

This concept of the organizational context and its complexity gave birth to many diverse viewpoints on leadership and spurred pivotal studies of leadership. One of the more important advances was evidentiary support for the idea that multiple styles, approaches, and methods could provide effective leadership. Contingency or situational leadership theories, which postulate that there is not one single best way to lead and that good leadership depends on the situation, began to flourish. While the most significant theories surfaced in the 1960s, the full impact of the relevance of contingency and situational leadership continues to be felt today.

Stogdill (1975, 165) goes further in suggesting that leaders are "not self-made and not a product of personality, drive, or ability." Bass

(2008, 85) states it simply: "The leader is a product of the situation and circumstances." Hughes, Ginnett, and Curphy (2015, 15) suggest an *interactional framework* approach to leadership. Essentially, this approach suggests that leadership is a function of three factors—the leader, the followers, and the situation they both face. Exhibit 2.2 provides a visual look at this concept.

Leadership style theories also began to surface during this time. The first variation of this theory, developed by Blake and Mouton (1964), is a simple two-factor concept of leadership that tried to identify what behaviors distinguished leaders from followers. They argue that leaders emphasize either people or tasks and results.

Similar to but more complex than the interactional framework view are contingency leadership theories, which gained a following through the work of Hersey and Blanchard (1969) and Fiedler (1986). These theories contend that different types of leaders are needed for different types of people and situations. As Hughes, Ginnett, and Curphy (2015, 525) explain, "In contingency leadership, leadership effectiveness is maximized when leaders correctly make their behaviors *contingent* on certain situational and follower characteristics."

Another way to view the fact that there is *not* "one best approach" to leading is to consider that the most effective leaders are those who can adapt. In our book, Garman and I (2015, 185) list adaptability as

Exhibit 2.2 Interactive Framework of Leadership

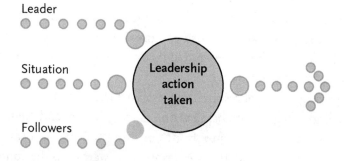

one of our critical leadership competencies (Dye and Garman 2015, 185). We posit that being adaptable "requires leaders to take a more active role in planning for their interactions, reflecting on how they went, and doing so on a consistent basis." Note also that this often means that leaders who lack the adaptability competency may be quite effective in certain situations but fail in different situations.

Because the foundation and essentials of situational and contingency theories still have great applicability today, exploring them in depth is useful. By using the framework of the leader, the followers, and the situation, the complexities of leadership can be fully examined.

The Leader

Much of leadership understanding and thought concentrates on the leader. To grow and develop, leaders ask these questions: "What should I be, what do I need to know, and what must I be able to do?" This principle is well illustrated through the US Army leadership paradigm (Hesselbein and Shinseki 2004). Certainly, the concept of traits from trait theory has logical applicability here. Essentially, the question to be answered is, "What does the leader need to be able to do (as a result of what she is and knows)?"

The Followers

The reality is that much of leadership depends on the followers. This idea is even more true today, given the nature of the workforce. What are the capabilities of the followers? How personally motivated are they to work toward the leader's vision? What is the complexity of the tasks to be handled by the followers? What are the interpersonal relationships between the followers and the leader? What are the power and ability of the leader to reward and reinforce their behavior?

A growing body of research suggests that the way to influence—and to lead—begins with being warm. Cuddy, Kohut, and Neffinger (2013, 56) argue for the importance of using warmth as a starting point in enhancing leadership and state that "warmth is the conduit of influence: It facilitates trust and the communication and absorption of ideas." Many believe that trust is a prerequisite of effective leadership and, essentially, requires the leader to connect with the followers. Building trust requires a demonstration of caring for others and a willingness and ability to help them.

A secondary but important consideration is that practically everyone who is a leader is also a follower. Almost every leader has a boss, including CEOs who report to boards of trustees. Thus, all leaders have the chance to reflect on followership. Moreover, many leaders view leadership from the perspective of how *they* themselves react and behave toward their leaders.

The Situation

Though Hersey, Blanchard, and Natemeyer (1979) built the foundations of the theory early on, Hersey, Blanchard, and Johnson (2007) further developed a model called situational leadership, which proposes four styles of leadership often labeled *telling, selling, participating*, and *delegating*.

This model suggests that leaders react to both tasks and people relationships. Moreover, leaders exhibit one of four styles of leadership:

1. *High emphasis on tasks and low emphasis on relationships*— often called a "telling" style; taken to extremes, represents an autocratic leader

2. *High emphasis on tasks and high emphasis on relationships*—a "selling" style; involves persuasion

3. *High emphasis on relationships and low emphasis on tasks*—a participative style; little direction given to followers

4. *Low emphasis on relationships and low emphasis on tasks*—a delegating style

Note that all four styles may have their place in leadership. For example, if the followers are resistant or unskilled, the leader may need to be much more directive in style. If the followers are highly motivated, capable, and skilled, the leader's style should be much more delegating in nature. A better understanding of their employees and the nature of the work to be accomplished will help leaders better adapt their styles of leadership to fit the situation.

Along these lines, Northouse (2016, 93) suggests that for a leader to be effective, he must determine the best course of action by evaluating his "followers and assessing how competent and committed they are to perform a given goal." In addition, according to Kaifi and colleagues (2014, 30), the "three core competencies of a situational leader are: diagnosing, flexibility, and partnering." Perhaps the most important learning point of this idea is the necessity of leaders being skilled and perceptive listeners who are constantly scanning the environment to discern the issues and concerns of the organization and its people.

From a practical viewpoint, the situational approach to leadership indicates that (1) leaders need to know themselves well through self-awareness, (2) leaders need to know their followers through listening and perception, and (3) leaders need to know conditions and circumstances by surveying and understanding their organizations.

Transformational (1970s Through the Present)

Burns (1978) and Bass (2008) presented the theory of *transformational leadership*. Much of the theory reflects the belief that followers want to be engaged in the vision for the organization. They need to understand—and subscribe to—a path for the future. Through what some describe as charismatic leadership, the leader motivates or influences followers to work toward strategic changes. Although no direct linkage is made in the literature, transformational leadership theory may have played some role in the development of the employee engagement movement.

Some would posit that transformational leadership stands in contrast to *transactional leadership*, an older style in which leaders use rewards and punishments to get followers to work toward goals. According to Burns (1978, 26), transactional leadership is simply a situation in which "one person takes the initiative in making contact with others for the purpose of an exchange of valued things." For example, though the notion retains little empirical support, many leaders today believe that pay is one of the prime factors in convincing followers to follow. In contrast, transformational leadership is not based on the idea of power, authoritarian approaches, or command-and-control styles of leadership.

OTHER APPROACHES TO UNDERSTANDING LEADERSHIP THEORIES

Though the popularity of many theories has come and gone, several ideas have proven applicable beyond their eras. The next few theories have solid academic support and are also quite usable by practitioners on a day-by-day basis.

Defining Leadership as a Process

In *Organizational Behavior*, Kreitner and Kinicki (2012, 31) describe leadership as "a social influence process in which the leader seeks the voluntary participation of subordinates in an effort to reach organizational goals."

This definition is true in three ways:

1. Leadership is a process because it takes place over a period, with a beginning and an end. Usually, the end is the point when leadership's effectiveness may be ascertained.

2. Leadership does not mean intimidation of followers into participation. Some healthcare "leaders" coerce "volunteers" to help them accomplish goals, but this technique is never acceptable and is highly unethical.

3. Leadership moves toward achievement or is progress driven, which is another symbol of effectiveness.

Uhl-Bien (2006, 655) expands on the process approach by suggesting that "relationships—rather than authority, superiority, or dominance—appear to be key to new forms of leadership." She further indicates that the study of leadership needs to "consider processes that are not just about the quality of the relationship or even the type of relationship, but rather about the social dynamics by which leadership relationships form and evolve in the workplace."

Path-Goal Theory

This school of thought purports that leaders must have versatility and be adaptable to various types of followers, organizations, and occurrences and view leadership as a process that moves along a path toward a goal. It has great merit and is one of the most validated theories of leadership. Vroom (1964) originated the idea with the *expectancy theory* of leadership, which, not unlike transactional leadership theory, posits that followers act in certain ways because they expect a certain outcome. House (1971) expanded the expectancy theory, and it became known as *path-goal leadership*. Exhibit 2.3 shows the simplicity of this model.

House (1971, 326) states that supervisors have influence over such factors as "financial increases, promotion, assignment of more interesting tasks, or opportunities for personal growth and development." Not surprisingly, many leaders view their oversight of these factors as critical in their ability to lead by "control."

Defining Leadership Comprehensively

Ralph Stogdill (1984) wrote what may be the most comprehensive treatise on leadership, *Stogdill's Handbook of Leadership*. In the book, he argues that leadership is any of the following:

Exhibit 2.3 Factors Influencing Goal Achievement: Path-Goal Theory of Leadership

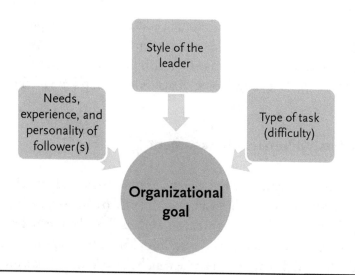

- A focus on team processes
- Personality and its effects
- The art of inducing compliance
- The exercise of influence
- An act that results in others acting or responding in a shared direction
- A form of persuasion
- A power relation
- An instrument of goal achievement
- An emerging effect of interaction
- A differentiated role
- The initiation of structure

Furthermore, Stogdill believes that interaction between members of a team occurs when one team member modifies the motivation or competencies of others in the team. Leaders are "agents of change, persons whose acts affect other people more than other people's acts affect them" (Stogdill 1984, 86).

This comprehensive catalog of definitions serves as a checklist, pointing leaders to areas for improvement. Although the comprehensive theory explains the technical aspects of leadership, it ignores its art and spirituality. Doing so makes leadership seem mechanical.

Leadership Versus Management

The two terms *leadership* and *management* are often used interchangeably. Strictly speaking, this is an error. It leads to confusion, and many popular books today suggest that all workers should aspire to be leaders. In his book *A Force for Change*, John Kotter (1990) proposes that leadership is different from management because leadership is a process that focuses on making organizational changes, while management is primarily concerned with control and results. In contrasting leadership with management, Kotter (2001) notes that "both are necessary for success in an increasingly complex and volatile environment."

Although Kotter agrees that both responsibilities are important, he views leaders as the stimuli behind their organization's adoption of—and adaptation to—improved processes. As a result, many of his readers are convinced that being a leader is preferable to being a manager. But a full analysis of leadership and management should clearly show that organizations do need both to be successful. Moreover, most leaders manage and most managers lead.

COMPETENCY-BASED LEADERSHIP

The various definitions under Stogdill's comprehensive theory support the view that leadership is enabled by a set of competencies. The *competency theory*, which has gained a significant following in the past decade, suggests that leaders must demonstrate knowledge, skills, and abilities in several areas, such as communications and business. Competency-based leadership also means that the key competencies required for specific roles in a corporate culture are identified and prioritized by organizations when they engage in recruitment, make decisions regarding promotions, and develop leaders.

For example, a chief financial officer will require competencies different from those of a chief medical officer. A formal, structured organization requires different competencies than does a more laid-back environment. In *Exceptional Leadership,* Garman and I contend that "competencies work so well [because] they are so practical" (Dye and Garman 2015, xxiv). We further state that the competency theory leads to "a better understanding of the key qualities that drive highly effective leadership."

The Institute of Medicine's (2003) report *Health Professions Education: A Bridge to Quality* gave impetus to the competency movement in healthcare. The report observes the insufficient number of tools for assessing the proficiency of healthcare professionals and suggests a set of core competencies designed to improve quality of care. In addition, the Healthcare Leadership Alliance—a collaboration among five healthcare professional associations—issued a competency tool with 300 competencies (for more information, see www.healthcareleadershipalliance.org). In the past several years, many other competency frameworks have been developed for both healthcare management practice and education (Stefl 2008).

By providing specific examples, competency theory enables leaders to "see" the behaviors ideal for competent leadership. For instance, it describes and explains the traits or competencies of an effective communicator. Moreover, the competency approach promotes the development and use of indicators that can measure the strength or weakness of a given competency.

Because many models include 80 or more competencies, picking out the competencies critical for effective leadership becomes a challenge. The book *Exceptional Leadership* lays out the 16 key competencies that distinguish great leadership from good leadership. See exhibit 2.4 for the Dye–Garman Leadership Competency Model.

Exhibit 2.4 Dye–Garman Leadership Competency Model

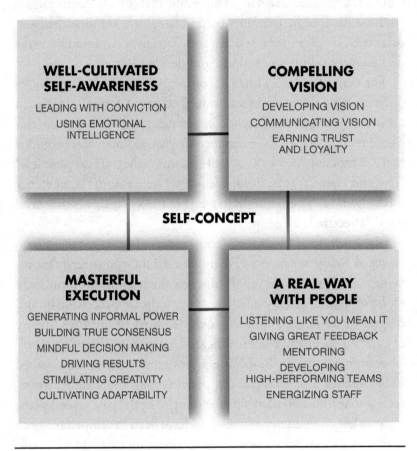

WELL-CULTIVATED SELF-AWARENESS

LEADING WITH CONVICTION

USING EMOTIONAL INTELLIGENCE

COMPELLING VISION

DEVELOPING VISION

COMMUNICATING VISION

EARNING TRUST AND LOYALTY

SELF-CONCEPT

MASTERFUL EXECUTION

GENERATING INFORMAL POWER

BUILDING TRUE CONSENSUS

MINDFUL DECISION MAKING

DRIVING RESULTS

STIMULATING CREATIVITY

CULTIVATING ADAPTABILITY

A REAL WAY WITH PEOPLE

LISTENING LIKE YOU MEAN IT

GIVING GREAT FEEDBACK

MENTORING

DEVELOPING HIGH-PERFORMING TEAMS

ENERGIZING STAFF

Source: Reprinted from Dye and Garman (2015).

Leadership Viewed by Psychology

While some leadership books and articles steer clear of the field of psychology, I believe that approach is quite short-sighted. Psychology provides much research-based literature on and support for the principles of leadership. Hogan (2009, slide 3) sums up the issue quite effectively, stating, "The fundamental problems in life concern 'getting along' and 'getting ahead'—developing relationships and developing a career. These themes exist in a state of tension. We resolve these problems during social interaction. Some people are better at this than others, and they tend to move into leadership positions."

Effective leaders consider their own personalities and the impact they have on their followers.

The Five-Factor Model of Personality

The *five-factor model of personality* has great similarities to some traditional trait theories. Using the acronym OCEAN (O = Openness to experience, C = Conscientiousness, E = Extraversion, A = Agreeableness, N = Neuroticism), the model purports to describe personality holistically. Likely profiles of highly effective and less effective leaders might look like those in exhibit 2.5. Applied to leadership, the model implies that effective leaders have broad interests and knowledge, are orderly and task focused, are extraverts who get along well with

---

Exhibit 2.5 Leader Profiles Using the Five-Factor Model

Highly Effective Leader

- Openness: very open to experiences
- Conscientiousness: very conscientious
- Extraversion: extraverted
- Agreeableness: agreeable, easy to get along with
- Neuroticism: calm and emotionally resilient

Less Effective Leader

- Openness: reserved and quiet, not comfortable out in front
- Conscientiousness: disorganized
- Extraversion: introverted
- Agreeableness: lacks warmth, can be hostile
- Neuroticism: Anxious, impatient

---

people, are positive in outlook, and have good emotional intelligence. While the five-factor model can be a great tool for enhancing self-awareness, Sokolov and I note that it is "not invincible. For example, many people who are naturally introverted are able to behaviorally exhibit strong extraverted skills that allow them to function as effective leaders" (Dye and Sokolov 2013, 153). Regarding the introverted-extraverted part of the model, Grant, Gino, and Hofman (2011, 528) write that "scholars have begun to question whether this conclusion [that extraverts have advantages as leaders] overstates the benefits of extraversion in leadership roles and overlooks the costs." It is interesting to note how so many discussions of leadership ultimately return to the situational or contingency theory viewpoint.

A grounded understanding of personality through the evidence presented in the field of psychology is critical. Hughes, Ginnett, and Curphy (2015, 189) state, "Given the accelerated pace of change in most organizations today, leaders will likely have even more unfamiliar and ambiguous situations in the future. Therefore, personality traits may play an increasingly important role in a leader's behavior." And Wallington (2003, 12) argues, "The dictionary definition of personality is the collection of emotional and behavioral traits that characterize a person. That is, your personality is how you present yourself to the world. It is how others see you. Is that important for leadership effectiveness? I think so. Your public persona is the catalyst for enrolling followers."

> Collectively, the research findings on leadership from all of these areas provide a picture of a process that is far more sophisticated and complex than the often simplistic view presented in some of the popular books on leadership.
>
> —Peter G. Northouse (2016)

A FINAL QUESTION—ASKED AND ANSWERED

Are leaders born or are leaders made? This question is posed throughout this book. Exhibit 2.6 summarizes the issue from an academic perspective.

Exhibit 2.6 Are Leaders Born or Made?

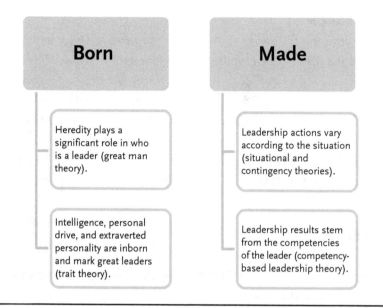

Born

- Heredity plays a significant role in who is a leader (great man theory).
- Intelligence, personal drive, and extraverted personality are inborn and mark great leaders (trait theory).

Made

- Leadership actions vary according to the situation (situational and contingency theories).
- Leadership results stem from the competencies of the leader (competency-based leadership theory).

CONCLUSION

The study of leadership from an academic perspective may often cause readers to feel as though they are going in circles. Yet the models and hypotheses provide great insight. The theories of contingency or situational leadership have great applicability to the practice of leadership today. With great changes occurring in society and the workplace, leaders must be able to interpret situations and deduce the best approach to take. Critical to this process are managing effectively (planning, organizing, staffing, controlling), having a firm understanding of the tasks or work to be completed, discerning how much guidance to provide to followers, and developing and leading teams. Understanding some of the research foundations of personality as it applies to leadership also gives leaders an enhanced self-awareness of their effectiveness.

Exercise

Exercise 2.1

Examine the following material and summarize how its conclusions apply to leadership effectiveness.

Francoeur, K. A. 2008. "The Relationship Between the Five-Factor Model of Personality and Leadership Preferences for Initiating Structure and Consideration." PhD diss., Indiana University of Pennsylvania. https://dspace.iup.edu/bitstream/handle/2069/99/Keith%20Francoeur.pdf.

REFERENCES

Barnard, C. I. 1938. *The Functions of the Executive*. Cambridge, MA: Harvard University Press.

Bass, B. M. 2008. *The Bass Handbook of Leadership: Theory, Research, and Managerial Applications*, 4th ed. New York: Free Press.

Blake, R. R., and J. S. Mouton. 1964. *The Managerial Grid: Key Orientations for Achieving Production Through People*. Houston, TX: Gulf Publishing.

Burns, J. M. 1978. *Leadership*. New York: Harper & Row.

Cuddy, A. J. C., M. Kohut, and J. Neffinger. 2013. "Connect, Then Lead." *Harvard Business Review*. Published July/August. https://hbr.org/2013/07/connect-then-lead.

Day, D. V., and J. Antonakis (eds.). 2012. *The Nature of Leadership*, 2nd ed. Los Angeles: SAGE Publications.

Dye, C. F., and A. N. Garman. 2015. *Exceptional Leadership: 16 Critical Competencies for Healthcare Executives*, 2nd ed. Chicago: Health Administration Press.

Dye, C. F., and J. J. Sokolov. 2013. *Developing Physician Leaders for Successful Clinical Integration*. Chicago: Health Administration Press.

Fiedler, F. E. 1986. "The Contribution of Cognitive Resources and Leader Behavior to Organizational Performance." *Journal of Applied Social Psychology* 16 (6): 532–45.

Gabor, A., and J. T. Mahoney. 2013. "Chester Barnard and the Systems Approach to Nurturing Organizations." In *The Oxford Handbook of Management Theorists*, edited by M. Witzel and M. Warner, 134–54. New York: Oxford University Press.

Grant, A. M., F. Gino, and D. A. Hofmann. 2011. "Reversing the Extraverted Leadership Advantage: The Role of Employee Proactivity." *Academy of Management Journal* 54 (3): 528–50.

Hersey, P., and K. H. Blanchard. 1969. "An Introduction to Situational Leadership." *Training and Development Journal* 23: 26–34.

Hersey, P., K. H. Blanchard, and D. E. Johnson. 2007. *Management of Organizational Behavior*, 9th ed. Boston: Pearson.

Hersey, P., K. H. Blanchard, and W. E. Natemeyer. 1979. "Situational Leadership, Perception, and the Impact of Power." *Group Organization Management* 4 (4): 418–28.

Hesselbein, F., and E. Shinseki. 2004. *Be, Know, Do: Leadership the Army Way: Adapted from the Official Army Leadership Manual*. San Francisco: Jossey-Bass.

Hogan, R. 2009. "Personality, Leadership and Organizational Effectiveness." Presentation at the International Personnel

Assessment Council Annual Conference on Personnel Assessment, Nashville, TN, September. http://annex.ipacweb.org/library/conf/09/hogan.pdf.

House, R. J. 1971. "A Path Goal Theory of Leader Effectiveness." *Administrative Science Quarterly* 16 (3): 321–39.

Hughes, R. L., R. C. Ginnett, and G. J. Curphy. 2015. *Leadership: Enhancing the Lessons of Experience*, 8th ed. Burr Ridge, IL: McGraw-Hill Education.

Institute of Medicine. 2003. *Health Professions Education: A Bridge to Quality*. Washington, DC: National Academies Press.

Kaifi, B. A., A. O. Noor, N.-L. Nguyen, W. Aslami, and N. M. Khanfar. 2014. "The Importance of Situational Leadership in the Workforce: A Study Based on Gender, Place of Birth, and Generational Affiliation." *Journal of Contemporary Management* 3 (2): 29–40.

Kotter, J. 2001. "What Leaders Really Do." *Harvard Business Review*. Published December. https://hbr.org/2001/12/what-leaders-really-do.

———. 1990. *A Force for Change: How Leadership Differs from Management*. New York: Free Press.

Kreitner, R., and A. Kinicki. 2012. *Organizational Behavior*, 10th ed. Burr Ridge, IL: McGraw-Hill Education.

Northouse, P. G. 2016. *Leadership: Theory and Practice*, 7th ed. Los Angeles: SAGE Publications.

Stefl, M. 2008. "Common Competencies for All Healthcare Managers: The Healthcare Leadership Alliance Model." *Journal of Healthcare Management* 53 (6): 360–74.

Stogdill, R. 1984. *Stogdill's Handbook of Leadership: A Survey of Theory and Research*. New York: Free Press.

————. 1975. "The Evolution of Leadership Theory." *Academy of Management Proceedings* 1: 4–6.

Uhl-Bien, M. 2006. "Relational Leadership Theory: Exploring the Social Processes of Leadership and Organizing." *Leadership Quarterly* 17 (6): 654–76.

Vroom, V. H. 1964. *Work and Motivation*. San Francisco: Jossey-Bass.

Wallington, P. 2003. "How Personality Plays into Leadership." *CIO*. Published January 15. www.cio.com/article/2440255/careers-staffing/how-personality-plays-into-leadership.html.

SUGGESTED READING

US Army. 2008. "Situational Leadership." In *Foundations of Leadership: MSL II*, 34–35. New York: Custom Publishing. www.mc.edu/rotc/files/9213/1471/9571/MSL_202_L09b_Situational_Leadership.pdf.

CHAPTER 3

Is the Popular Leadership Literature Worthless?

*Ultimately, then, good leadership is
the key to organizational effectiveness.*

—Robert Hogan and Robert B. Kaiser (2005)

THREE **CEO**s WERE discussing their investments in leadership development. The first said, "We've really turned the heat up this year. All our leaders are going through the 'Lead Like a Rock Star' development program. I know the title sounds off, but we found that rock stars shared several principles with strong leaders. They're very focused, they practice a lot, they're accustomed to being under the bright lights, and they're always preparing for the next big show. According to our consultant, leadership is a lot like that. He has assessments and modules built around the idea, and our leaders are really loving the program."

The second CEO replied, "Sounds odd, but I guess I'll give you the benefit of the doubt! Four years ago we started our 'Journey to Change' program. It's based on the book by Fred Futures, *Be Prepared for Your Journey*. There's a lot of reflective meditation in the various exercises, and our leaders are asked to do a lot of journaling and reflective work."

The third CEO replied, "Well, I guess our program is pretty different. It doesn't sound as jazzy as both of yours. We use several faculty members from the local university and we have some of the National Hospital Association keynote speakers come to us. We built the program around a lot of academic literature and use real-world projects that we assign to our leaders. They work in teams and function a lot like internal consultants. We started a similar program for our physician leaders last year."

ANY STUDY OF leadership that neglects or overlooks the popular literature on the subject is doing a disservice to students of leadership. For purposes of our discussion in this chapter, the phrase *popular leadership literature* comprises books that are read zealously by practitioners of leadership. Many of their readers become staunch followers—fans of a sort.

Bookstores are filled with leadership texts that become so celebrated that many practicing leaders fail to challenge the soundness and logic of their premises. I often think of these titles as "airport leadership books." Many individuals purchase them in airports, apparently hoping that they are only a plane ride away from leadership perfection.

Simply put, some of the popular leadership literature is full of holes, lacking substantiation or evidence for the assertions made.

On the other hand, much of the academic literature reviewed in chapter 2 is, admittedly, hard to read and often full of tedious and mind-numbing statistics. Many of these articles appear in refereed professional journals and are not read by—or even available to—the average person in the C-suite. This literature does not appear in the airport bookstores or on Amazon.com and may be difficult to find, and its largest group of readers is currently in graduate school. Moreover, Hogan and Kaiser (2005, 171) state that the "academic tradition is a collection of dependable empirical nuggets, but it is also a collection of decontextualized facts that do not add up to a persuasive account of leadership." Simply put, it cannot compete successfully with the popular literature.

What leader has not heard of *The 7 Habits of Highly Successful People* (Covey 2013), *Good to Great* (Collins 2001), *The Five Dysfunctions of a Team: A Leadership Fable* (Lencioni 2002), *Who Moved My Cheese?* (Johnson and Blanchard 1998), or *Crucial Conversations* (Patterson et al. 2011)?

While commercial books may offer excellent lessons and great suggestions, the true student of leadership should always exercise caution and thoughtfulness when reading them. Look for evidence backing the assertions made in these publications. Are their ideas logical? Are they based on documented facts? Look to the questions posed in the next sections to challenge the premises of the popular leadership literature. The primary intent of this chapter is to get readers to be more judicious with the material they read, study, and adopt.

> The consuming interest in leadership and how to make it better has spawned a plethora of books, blogs, TED talks, and commentary. Unfortunately, these materials are often wonderfully disconnected from organizational reality and, as a consequence, useless for sparking improvement. Maybe that's one reason the enormous resources invested in leadership development have produced so few results.
>
> —Jeffrey Pfeffer (2016)

Is It Supported by Evidence?

Hogan and Kaiser (2005, 171) describe many commercial books as part of the "troubadour tradition." They state that "despite its popularity, the troubadour tradition is a vast collection of opinions with very little supporting evidence; it is entertaining but unreliable." Are the books filled with anecdotal observations? How reliable—and statistically valid—are their claims? What is the academic background or professional experience of the author(s)?

While it is not in the purview of this book to expound extensively on evidence-based practice, doing so has become common in healthcare. The medical profession has profoundly changed in response to A. L. Cochrane's 1972 book *Effectiveness and Efficiency*, which condemns the lack of reliable evidence behind many widely accepted healthcare interventions.

The business world has caught up with this trend. Pfeffer and Sutton (2006) wrote an excellent *Harvard Business Review* article titled "Evidence-Based Management." It discusses the problem of "repeatedly adopting, then abandoning, one ill-supported business fad after another." Moreover, they point out the existence of "a huge body of peer-reviewed studies—literally thousands . . . that although routinely ignored, provide simple and powerful advice about how to run organizations." And Rousseau (2006, 256) writes about "the failure of organizations and managers to base practices on best available evidence."

Readers should be mindful that solid evidence excludes such things as opinion, bias, hearsay, and fallacy.

Is It Applicable?

After determining that there is valid support for its premise, perhaps the next best way to evaluate popular leadership literature is to test its applicability—for example, by asking if Covey's (2013) seven habits support effective leadership. Most practicing leaders would argue that these principles do.

Consider one theory that has been broadly questioned in practice: strengths-based leadership, popularized by the Rath and Conchie (2013) book *Strengths Based Leadership*. Although the book is allegedly supported by research from Gallup, Kaplan and Kaiser (2009) argue that "it turns out you can take strengths too far" by failing to recognize and work on weaknesses. They suggest that the strengths-based approach can be overused and can greatly harm a leader. Chamorro-Premuzic (2016) also shows that the strengths approach means that "people get feedback on their relative strengths and weaknesses but cannot tell how they stack up against the competition—i.e., other people."

How to Deal with Academic Literature

Readers are encouraged to try a blend of both popular and academic literature. Although it can be dry, Brenner (2004, 99) explains that "scholarly discourse, especially written scholarly discourse, has a certain format. It is supposed to be factual and dry, 'objective,' or at least relatively clean of personal influence. It is supposed to contain extensive references to previous and current chains of learning." In other words, academic literature is dry by design, in an effort to avoid the very trendiness that seems to characterize popular literature.

Be mindful, when reading the academic literature, that its focus can be quite narrow. Many leaders prefer to read broader and more all-encompassing material on leadership. Much of the academic literature provides a deep, drill-down analysis of one aspect of leadership. This exhaustive nature makes it arduous and mind-numbing to read.

The Benefits of Popular Leadership Books

So, should students of leadership and practitioner leaders ignore the popular literature? Simply stated, no. In fact, some of the popular literature is actually supported by academic literature—the writers simply do not provide a large amount of scholarly content to avoid becoming dull and uninteresting. Many readers who would otherwise be bored to tears by typical journal articles and research-heavy books tend to be enthusiastically inspired by the precepts in the popular leadership literature. These readers then put the principles to work and often become more effective leaders as a result. Healthcare organizations sometimes build programs around these books, such as a communication program based on Patterson and colleagues' *Crucial Conversations* (2011).

The pros and cons of academic literature and popular literature are summarized in exhibit 3.1.

> Being an expert on leadership research is neither necessary nor sufficient for being a good leader.
>
> —Richard L. Hughes, Robert C. Ginnett, and Gordon J. Curphy (2015)

Exhibit 3.1 Pros and Cons of Academic and Popular Leadership Literature

Popular Leadership Literature		Academic Leadership Literature	
Pros	Cons	Pros	Cons
Easy to read	Conclusions may not be supported by evidence	Discussion is focused	Tedious to read—can be boring, repetitive, and uninspiring
Some premises are actually supported by solid research (although not always clearly stated)	May not fit situation or group of followers	Information is supported by evidence	
Examples drawn from real experience	May grossly oversimplify the practice of leadership	Information is not tied to the popularity of an individual author	
Accessible to leadership audience			Not easily accessible to leadership audience

Leadership Skill Theories and Competency Models

Skills-based leadership is one theory of leadership that has its roots in both academic and popular literature. Recently this theory has partially morphed into a competency-based view of leadership.

Mumford and colleagues (2000) write that, rather than emphasize what leaders do, the skills approach regards capabilities as what make effective leadership possible. Essentially, this means that leadership can be developed over time—it can be learned. Moreover, it suggests that if individuals are capable of learning, they can be leaders.

As Avolio, Walumbwa, and Weber (2009, 426) note, "Another very promising area of research that has not received sufficient attention in the leadership literature focuses on understanding what constitutes an individual's level of developmental readiness or one's capacity or motivational orientation to develop to one's full potential."

Garman and I propose in our book that the "answer to 'What makes a leader exceptional?' is simple: competencies. . . . We present a basic definition here. Leadership competencies are a set of professional and personal skills, knowledge, values, and traits that guide a leader's performance, behavior, interaction, and decisions" (Dye and Garman 2015, xiii). The Dye–Garman Leadership Competency Model is shown in exhibit 2.4.

CONCLUSION

Chapters 2 and 3 cover material that can fill a semester of a typical graduate-level leadership class. Certainly, academic and popular literature each has a place in the study of leadership. Be sure to challenge the popular leadership literature and not fall prey to leadership ideas that are not supported by facts and evidence.

Self-Evaluation Questions

❑ Have I ever become so enthralled with a book that I did not thoroughly assess its logic?

❑ Have I initiated programs that may be viewed negatively as the next program du jour?

❑ Am I guilty of following the newest management or leadership trends?

(continued)

(continued from previous page)

❑ Do I occasionally review the academic literature on leadership, or do I typically dismiss it as dry and boring?

❑ Are my bookshelves filled with partially read, popular leadership books that were once "hot" but have now lost their luster?

Exercises

Exercise 3.1

Read "What We Know About Leadership" by Hogan and Kaiser (2005). What is your impression of Hogan and Kaiser's (p. 171) "troubadour tradition" literature? To what extent does this article encourage you to read the classic "academic tradition" literature?

Hogan, R., and R. B. Kaiser. 2005. "What We Know About Leadership." *Review of General Psychology* 9 (2): 169–80.

The article is available online at http://psychology.illinoisstate.edu/ktschne/psy376/Hogan_Kaiser.pdf. A narrative review of the article can be found at www.peterberry.com.au/files/hogan_white_papers/what_we_know_about_leadership.pdf.

Exercise 3.2

Review the following webpage. What do you conclude about using caution when reading popular leadership books and articles?

McNamara, C. 2016. "Guidelines to Understand Literature on Leadership." Free Management Library. Accessed May 9. http://managementhelp.org/leadership/development/literature.htm.

REFERENCES

Avolio, B. J., F. O. Walumbwa, and T. J. Weber. 2009. "Leadership: Current Theories, Research, and Future Directions." *Annual Review of Psychology* 60: 421–49.

Brenner, A. 2004. *I Am . . .: Biblical Women Tell Their Own Stories.* Minneapolis, MN: Augsburg Fortress Publishers.

Chamorro-Premuzic, T. 2016. "Strengths-Based Coaching Can Actually Weaken You." *Harvard Business Review*. Published January 4. https://hbr.org/2016/01/strengths-based-coaching-can-actually-weaken-you.

Cochrane, A. L. 1972. *Effectiveness and Efficiency: Random Reflections on Health Services.* London: Nuffield Provincial Hospitals Trust. www.nuffieldtrust.org.uk/sites/files/nuffield/publication/Effectiveness_and_Efficiency.pdf.

Collins, J. 2001. *Good to Great: Why Some Companies Make the Leap . . . and Others Don't.* New York: HarperCollins.

Covey, S. R. 2013. *The 7 Habits of Highly Successful People: Powerful Lessons in Personal Change*, 25th anniversary ed. New York: Simon and Schuster.

Dye, C. F., and A. N. Garman. 2015. *Exceptional Leadership: 16 Critical Competencies for Healthcare Executives*, 2nd ed. Chicago: Health Administration Press.

Hogan, R., and R. B. Kaiser. 2005. "What We Know About Leadership." *Review of General Psychology* 9 (2): 169–80.

Hughes, R. L., R. C. Ginnett, and G. J. Curphy. 2015. *Leadership: Enhancing the Lessons of Experience*, 8th ed. Burr Ridge, IL: McGraw-Hill Education.

Johnson, S., and K. Blanchard. 1998. *Who Moved My Cheese? An A-Mazing Way to Deal with Change in Your Work and in Your Life.* New York: Putnam.

Kaplan, R. E., and R. B. Kaiser. 2009. "Stop Overdoing Your Strengths." *Harvard Business Review.* Published February. https://hbr.org/2009/02/stop-overdoing-your-strengths.

Lencioni, P. 2002. *The Five Dysfunctions of a Team: A Leadership Fable.* San Francisco: Jossey-Bass.

Mumford, M. D., S. J. Zaccaro, F. D. Harding, T. O. Jacobs, and E. A. Fleishman. 2000. "Leadership Skills for a Changing World: Solving Complex Social Problems." *Leadership Quarterly* 11 (1): 11–35.

Patterson, K., J. Grenny, R. McMillan, and A. Switzler. 2011. *Crucial Conversations: Tools for Talking When the Stakes Are High,* 2nd ed. New York: McGraw-Hill.

Pfeffer, J. 2016. "Getting Beyond the BS of Leadership Literature." *McKinsey Quarterly.* Published January. www.mckinsey.com/global-themes/leadership/getting-beyond-the-bs-of-leadership-literature.

Pfeffer, J., and R. I. Sutton. 2006. "Evidence-Based Management." *Harvard Business Review.* Published January. https://hbr.org/2006/01/evidence-based-management.

Rath, T., and B. Conchie. 2013. *Strengths Based Leadership: Great Leaders, Teams, and Why People Follow.* New York: Gallup Press.

Rousseau, D. M. 2006. "Is There Such a Thing as 'Evidence-Based Management'?" *Academy of Management Review* 31 (2): 256–69.

SUGGESTED READINGS

Rousseau, D. M. 2006. "Keeping an Open Mind about Evidence-Based Management: A Reply to Learmonth's Commentary." *Academy of Management Review* 31 (4): 1091–93.

Rousseau, D. M., and S. McCarthy. 2007. "Educating Managers from an Evidence-Based Perspective." *Academy of Management Learning and Education* 6 (1): 84–101.

CHAPTER 4

The Values-Based Definition

Leadership, simply put, is the ability to influence others.
Values-based leadership takes it to the next level. By word,
action, and example, values-based leaders seek to inspire and
motivate, using their influence to pursue what matters most.

—Harry Kraemer (2011)

A HEALTH SYSTEM CEO led a discussion on leadership with second-year health administration graduate students. He posed the following questions: "Was Hitler an effective leader? Was Stalin an effective leader? And note that I did call them leaders. And before you answer, consider the fact that there's a leadership book called *Leadership Secrets of Attila the Hun* that's been popular since the 1980s. So I will add another question: Was Attila the Hun an effective leader?"

He went on to say, "If the primary goal of leadership is to get results, didn't Hitler and Stalin and Attila get results? Is it not evident that many, many people followed each of them?"

He continued, "As leaders, are results all that matter? Is there something that makes us different from Hitler, Stalin, or Attila—or similar to them, for that matter? Does the concept of values come into play here? And can we even truly define values effectively when talking about leadership? Do some leaders have a set of values that is different from Hitler's? Is that a key deciding factor? If the answer is yes, then it would seem important—no, it would be *absolutely critical*—that as we study leadership, we must learn the role that values play in leadership."

AFTER LOOKING AT leadership from an academic perspective in chapter 2 and from a popular perspective in chapter 3, this chapter moves in a different direction. It provides the determinative foundation for the theme of this book—that is, internal values drive external behavior; effective leadership does, in fact, have a certain set of values; and those values drive the external behavior that helps make leaders effective. As stated in the preface, values come into play here.

But in establishing the definition of leadership for our purposes, we now add the requirement that effective leadership must have some beneficial good or purpose behind it. The vision must have a level of purity that benefits humankind.

For those of us who work in healthcare, serving in the field may be what many describe as the higher calling. The classic Robert Frost poem "The Road Not Taken" (see exhibit 4.1) underscores the conscious—and unusual—choice that exceptional leaders must make to live and lead according to their values. Their choices make all the difference, both in their lives and in the lives of those they serve.

> External factors, such as changing regulations or pressure to meet financial goals, can threaten to move even the most ethical leaders on a perilous journey toward unethical decisions.
>
> —Carson F. Dye and Brett D. Lee (2016)

BORN OR MADE? A VALUES-BASED RESPONSE

Chapter 2 reviews some theories that scholars have developed in response to the question, Are leaders born or made? I contend that

Exhibit 4.1 "The Road Not Taken" by Robert Frost

Two roads diverged in a yellow wood,
And sorry I could not travel both
And be one traveler, long I stood
And looked down one as far as I could
To where it bent in the undergrowth;

Then took the other, as just as fair,
And having perhaps the better claim,
Because it was grassy and wanted wear;
Though as for that the passing there
Had worn them really about the same,

And both that morning equally lay
In leaves no step had trodden black.
Oh, I kept the first for another day!
Yet knowing how way leads on to way,
I doubted if I should ever come back.

I shall be telling this with a sigh
Somewhere ages and ages hence:
Two roads diverged in a wood, and I—
I took the one less traveled by,
And that has made all the difference.

Source: Frost (2016).

1. leadership is both inherent and learned, and
2. leadership values and skills are interrelated. One cannot exist without the other.

Numerous studies suggest that many leadership skills and traits are the result of heredity (Hughes, Ginnett, and Curphy 2015). In this vein, so-called born leaders tend to develop certain values and exhibit strong leadership characteristics and skills *early* in life. Many managers, executives, and consultants—including me—hold the belief that those who are not born leaders must cultivate these values to enhance their leadership capabilities. Essentially, they have the possibility of learning behaviors or skills (read "competencies") that make them effective leaders.

What definitive characteristics differentiate strong leaders from weak leaders? What traits drive the behavior of effective leaders? What qualities do successful leaders possess that average leaders do not have? The only answer is having the appropriate leadership values.

WHAT ARE VALUES?

Values are ingrained principles that guide behaviors and thoughts. They are formed early in life and are likely correlated somewhat to heredity. They do develop more deeply with experiences and usually do not change much during a lifetime. As a moral framework, values help an individual analyze options, make decisions during times of stress, and rise above difficult or unexpected situations. Values are not necessarily all positive, however. Exhibit 4.2 provides an analogy for understanding how values are connected with and drive behaviors and thoughts.

Everyone has values, but those values differ from person to person. Some people have values that affect their leadership effectiveness. For example, Leader A highly regards being around other people, while Leader B highly regards being alone. Because Leader A spends time with others, she is more exposed to others' ideas and practices. She can learn from this exposure and, in the process, develop an appreciation for and openness to different experiences. Leader B's values, on the other hand, may not be as conducive to leadership improvement because he is isolated from the opinions and experiences of others. The real advantage of positive values depends on the degree to which a person allows these values to influence her development.

Sarros and Santora (2001, 7) state that "executives whose values are grounded in fundamental human virtues such as benevolence

Exhibit 4.2 The Iceberg Analogy of Leadership Values

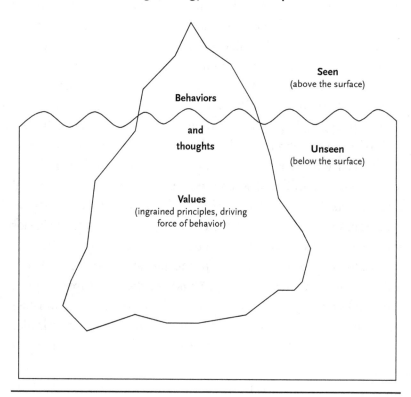

and honesty, but who also retain a need for personal gratification and success, are closely associated with transformational behaviors."

Personal and Team Values

One of the foundational precepts of this book is that there are both personal and team values that drive appropriate and effective leadership behavior. Learning these can make it easier to adopt effective leadership behavior.

Personal values affect how a leader perceives and is perceived by others. If leadership is a "social influence process," as Kreitner and Kinicki

(2012, 34) suggest, then values can make an impact—negatively or positively—on this process. A leader is most influential when his followers know what he stands for because followers are clear on whether they can relate to the leader's ideals. This concept is illustrated whenever any new leader assumes a new leadership position. Practically all new leaders exert great effort to ensure that those in their new organizations know where they stand *personally*. One CEO remarks, "I spend much of my first 90 days helping people to learn—and understand—my personal history and style—this is who I am, why I am, and what I stand for. That way they will have a better understanding of the changes I will make." The same can be said of CEOs when they seek buy-in from organizational stakeholders. Lee and I state it clearly: "Executives must develop an understanding of leadership that includes a grasp of how their behavior influences the environment around them" (Dye and Lee 2016, 14).

In addition, personal values guide the interactions between a leader and her followers, serving as the "fluid" of the social interchange. Under the contingency theory, in which a leader considers all variables before making a decision and moving forward, an effective leader relies on her values to steer her toward the most appropriate action.

The *influence* dimension of leadership requires the leader to have an impact on the lives of those being led. To make a change in other people carries with it an enormous ethical burden and responsibility. Because leaders usually have more power and control than [do their] followers, they also have more responsibility to be sensitive to how their leadership affects followers' lives.

—Peter G. Northouse (2016)

Team values are commonly referred to using the French phrase *esprit de corps*, or *spirit of the group*. They serve as a bond that connects and links team members. These values guide the behaviors, decisions, and actions of team members. They also set the standards for how members interact with each other and work together, given that each member holds differing personal values that could cause conflicts in the group. In an organization, team values are often, if not always, tied to the mission of the enterprise. For example, if the mission is to serve those in need, regardless of their ability to pay, the team values will likely include community service, respect for diversity, accountability, and open communication—not pursuit of profits or one-upmanship.

Exhibit 4.3 Personal Values Versus Team Values

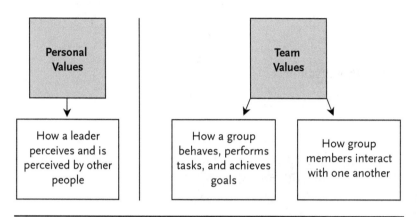

Personal and team values contribute to leadership effectiveness. Exhibit 4.3 provides a distinction between these two types of values.

Values That Drive Behaviors

At the time of this writing, a Google search for "list of values" provided more than a billion results. Refining that to "list of leadership values" yielded 241 million results. Steve Pavlina (2004) offers a frequently cited "short" list of 418 values. Here are just a few:

- Acceptance
- Accessibility
- Accomplishment
- Accountability
- Care
- Compassion
- Community
- Empathy
- Fairness

- Honesty
- Justice
- Perseverance
- Resolve
- Thoughtfulness
- Truth
- Zeal

Reviewing such lists can be an illuminating exercise for leadership students and practitioners alike.

Sample Personal Values Statement

This real-life example of a personal values statement is provided courtesy of a healthcare executive who wishes to remain anonymous. She shared this with me as we discussed values-based leadership.

I really do have a personal values statement, and I have actually written it out. I compare my leadership to an actual journey, and I see my values as the guiding essentials on that journey. Each element has a name and includes various thoughts about that value.

Wind behind my back. I always want to journey to see new things and to make improvements.

Compass that points true north. I want to let the deeper forces within me that developed through my early years continue to guide me. Therefore, I do a lot of reflection while I am on the trail.

People on the trail with me. I have teams. Even though they may report to me, I view them as peers on this journey. The fact is that others help make me look good.

Sunshine ahead of me. I walk toward the light. I don't mean this in a religious sense, but this speaks to my interest in transparency and doing the right things.

Share lunch during the trip. I am grateful to live in a wealthy nation and work in a well-paid career. I try to give back as much as I can—not only to charities but to the workers around me.

My head is often down. This speaks to both my humility as well as to my keen focus on detail. Do it right, and do it right the first time.

Always carry a book. I have always been a lifelong learner. Books are gifts that broaden your view of the trail.

A song to sing. This is the cheesy part. I grew up listening to the rock band Journey. Their song "Don't Stop Believin'" is the song I sing on the trail. To me it means being positive about change and the work we all do.

An excellent example of a corporate leadership values statement is provided in exhibit 4.4. This text from Bayer could easily be used as an exemplary model for an individual leadership values statement as well.

Values Espoused in This Book

While the following values, which underlie the content of this book, may not precisely fit under a traditional definition of values, I contend that they are critical for effective leadership:

- Respect
- Ethical behavior
- Integrity
- Interpersonal connection
- Servant leadership
- Desire to make a change
- Commitment
- Emotional intelligence
- Cooperation and sharing

- Cohesiveness and collaboration
- Trust
- Conflict management

The first three values must be strong in the complex world of healthcare. Respecting everyone, practicing ethical behavior, and possessing high integrity provide a firm foundation for those who lead in a field that cares for people in times of great need.

Interpersonal connection and servant leadership are logically tied to what is done in a service business such as healthcare. I am struck by how many leaders in healthcare list these as two of the more important considerations for effective leadership. Exhibit 4.5 explores some of the wisdom of Richard L. Hughes, Robert C.

Exhibit 4.4 Bayer Leadership and Integrity Values

Leadership
- Be passionate for people and performance
- Show personal drive, inspire and motivate others
- Be accountable for actions and results, successes and failures
- Treat others fairly and with respect
- Give clear, candid and timely feedback
- Manage conflicts constructively
- Create value for all our stakeholders

Integrity
- Be a role model
- Comply with laws, regulations and good business practices
- Trust others and build trustful relationships
- Be honest and reliable
- Listen attentively and communicate appropriately
- Ensure sustainability: balance short-term results with long-term requirements
- Care about people, safety, and the environment

Source: Reprinted with permission from Bayer (2016).

Exhibit 4.5 Hughes, Ginnett, and Curphy on Values-Based Leadership

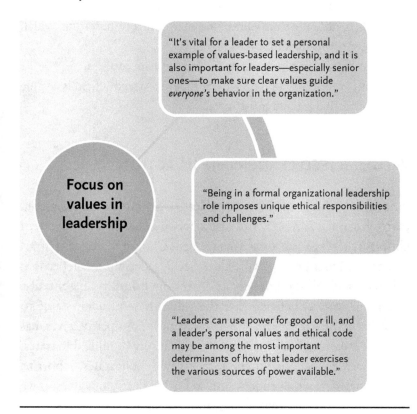

"It's vital for a leader to set a personal example of values-based leadership, and it is also important for leaders—especially senior ones—to make sure clear values guide *everyone's* behavior in the organization."

Focus on values in leadership

"Being in a formal organizational leadership role imposes unique ethical responsibilities and challenges."

"Leaders can use power for good or ill, and a leader's personal values and ethical code may be among the most important determinants of how that leader exercises the various sources of power available."

Source: Hughes, Ginnett, and Curphy (2015).

Ginnett, and Gordon J. Curphy, well-known authors in the leadership field, on the basic necessity of a good ethical foundation for those who exercise power.

The desire to make a change is a value that has always fueled healthcare. The improvement of quality and patient safety, the development of new technology, discoveries in pharmacology, new approaches to the care model, and the eradication of diseases such as cancer all emanate from this value. If clinicians are drawn to the field in part because they want to make a change, certainly their leaders should share this same value.

Healthcare is a demanding career—for leaders as well as for all who serve. Thus, commitment is a required value for leaders.

Emotional intelligence, cooperation and sharing, and cohesiveness and collaboration are values that matter in a team setting, which is where most leadership takes place.

Trust surfaces on practically all lists of leader values.

Finally, the ability to manage conflict in a stressful field is a value that all effective leaders must have.

VALUES-BASED LEADERSHIP IN ACTION

Putting the concept of values-based leadership into context is useful. Harry Kraemer, former CEO of Baxter and current Northwestern University Kellogg School of Management Clinical Professor of Strategy, presents four principles of values-based leadership: self-reflection, balance, true self-confidence, and genuine humility. Essentially, Kraemer (2011, 2) believes that the values-based leader is able to understand the self, can see situations from various perspectives, has a proper balance of self-confidence, and is truly humble. He states, "The way we treat customers, interact with colleagues, report to supervisors, deal with vendors, and so forth reflects our values. If we are not aware of those values, these interactions will not be effective."

Another way to better understand how values-based leadership works is to view it through three As: awareness, action, and achievement. A strong personal awareness of one's values and the values that drive highly effective leadership is a given for values-based leaders. One of the principles of this book is that internal values drive external behavior. If the values are the right ones, the resulting external behavior can serve to influence the actions needed to ultimately attain achievements that serve others. Exhibit 4.6 graphically portrays the three As.

Successful leaders share values with those they lead.

—Bernard M. Bass (2008)

Many executives who have read the earlier editions of this book have mentioned the uniqueness of viewing leadership from the lens of values. Yes,

Exhibit 4.6 Three As of Values-Based Leadership

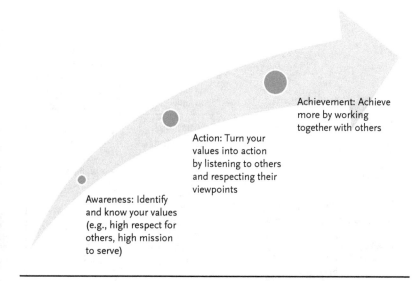

Achievement: Achieve more by working together with others

Action: Turn your values into action by listening to others and respecting their viewpoints

Awareness: Identify and know your values (e.g., high respect for others, high mission to serve)

many aspects of leadership are soft; many do not easily lend themselves to quantitative proof. Yet this softer side often makes the difference. Using a values-based approach to studying leadership is an excellent way to maximize understanding.

FOUR STAGES OF LEARNING AND MASTERY

Highly effective leaders are always interested in learning and enhancing their leadership competencies. Values enable them to go through the stages of leadership growth. Following is a description of each stage (also see exhibit 4.7).

Stage 1: Unconscious Incompetence

You don't know that you don't know. This stage is the most difficult for many leaders because they are unaware of their own mistakes

Exhibit 4.7 Learning and Mastery Process

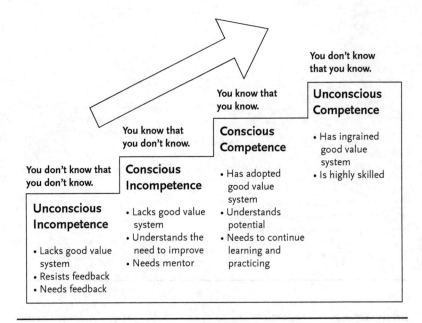

and flaws. Often, they work in successful organizations and do not even consider whether problems with their leadership skills might exist. Leaders most likely to be at this level are those who have not started to develop appropriate leadership values or may be highly resistant to the input and feedback of others. As a result, they need training and awareness to enhance their self-understanding.

> Moral leadership requires professional leaders to understand that it does matter that they like what they see in the mirror. It requires leaders to do, not just think of, what is right.
>
> —Elizabeth J. Forrestal and Leigh W. Cellucci (2016)

Stage 2: Conscious Incompetence

You know that you don't know. Although this stage is the most important step toward learning, it can be the most challenging because sometimes you have to lose your job before you realize that your performance needs work. For others, this realization is a gradual process and may come as the result of the influence of a strong mentor or coach and a sincere desire to grow and improve.

Stage 3: Conscious Competence

You know that you know. Some leaders are neither born nor strong, but at this stage, they start developing and honing their potential. Such leaders work hard to put into practice appropriate skills, but they sometimes fail because the skills are not part of their natural thinking habits yet.

Stage 4: Unconscious Competence

You don't know that you know. This stage is the ultimate level of leadership development because the activities here flow smoothly with neither great force nor hesitation. Leaders at this level seem to be naturals at their trade. Unconscious competence is truly descriptive of a born leader.

VALUES-BASED LEADERSHIP THEORY

One solid theory of leadership is that it is values-based. Copeland (2014, 130), in her excellent literature review of values-based leadership theory, states that "history has demonstrated repeatedly that leaders [who] lack ethical and value-based dimensions can have serious adverse consequences on their followers, their organizations, our nation and the world." George (2004) and Muscat and Whitty (2009) also specifically discuss values-based leadership.

Effective leadership is based on three factors: heredity, values, and competencies. As explained earlier, heredity in this context is the view that all persons are born with inherent characteristics (some have more than others) that enable them to practice leadership at some level of proficiency. Thus, the precept that leaders are born does carry logical support. The *values-based theory* of leadership posits that individuals develop certain (positive) values and behavioral skills or competencies that facilitate their practice of leadership—that is, leaders can also learn leadership.

But an individual must *desire* to be in a leadership position. Not everyone wants to be a leader. Many professionals in healthcare—particularly clinicians (e.g., physicians, nurses, pharmacists, therapists)—prefer to remain in clinical roles. As a result, they may not seek formal leadership positions. Certainly, they may act or serve as leaders within their clinical positions, but not consistently as full-time leaders do. Thus, motivation must be present for humans to engage in a particular behavior.

No matter the person's hereditary tendencies, values, and competencies, if the need or want (in other words, motivation) is absent, the person will not be a leader. Exhibit 4.8 presents this conceptually.

CONCLUSION

In summary, the concept of values is difficult to define. They are intensely personal, affecting individuals in profound ways. Despite some contributions to the literature over the past 20 years, values are not an area that many academics study. Perhaps it is because of the inspirational nature of values, which runs counter to the drily factual nature of academic inquiry. Perhaps it is because they are too deeply related to gestalt psychology, which is often considered a

Exhibit 4.8 Components of Effective Leadership

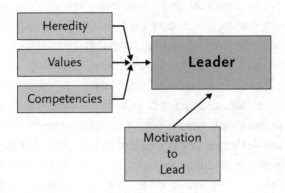

"soft" science. The origin of values is deeply personal, and each person's development of values is achieved though different experience and heredity. As much as we would like to define the concept absolutely, it will always remain abstract. Yet it is a critical component of effective leadership. Therefore, it is incumbent upon leaders to reflect on values and include them as part of our leadership studies.

Allowing positive values to be a primary influencer may be the most fundamental way that leaders can judge their own styles. Parts II and III of this book identify the values that guide leaders and team members. See appendix A for a professional and personal values assessment tool.

Self-Evaluation Questions

❑ What do I value? Do these values assist or hinder my leadership activities?

❑ Are my behaviors guided by personal values?

❑ What personal values of mine may conflict with my role and responsibilities as a leader?

❑ If I have written a narrative describing my leadership style, does it make reference to my personal values? Did I write this narrative to impress a search consultant or a potential employer, or did I do it to evaluate my strengths and weaknesses?

❑ Does my definition of leadership include some reference to values?

❑ What is my definition of leadership?

❑ List several successful healthcare leaders. What traits do they have in common? What values do they share?

❑ One Self-Evaluation Question in chapter 1 asks, "Do I view leadership as an act, a process, or a skill?" After reading chapter 4, how does my answer to this question differ?

Case and Exercise

Case 4.1

Three health system vice presidents (VPs) are discussing leadership over lunch. The first VP says, "Leadership is completely about relationships. It's about how you work with people and how you get to know them as individuals." The second VP replies, "I agree that people are important, but you can have a lot of happy people and not achieve any goals. That's not leadership in my book." The third VP comments, "You both have good points, but you're really missing the key of leadership—vision. A lot of what you're talking about is management. Leadership is developing a vision and getting the organization moving toward that vision."

You join these three VPs at the table, and they ask for your thoughts on this issue.

Case 4.1 Questions

1. Describe in detail how each VP's argument is right and wrong.

2. How might their differing viewpoints be melded together to provide a comprehensive and accurate definition of leadership?

Exercise 4.1

Find a list of values on the Internet. List the positive leadership actions that typically would emanate from these values.

REFERENCES

Bass, B. M. 2008. *The Bass Handbook of Leadership: Theory, Research, and Managerial Applications,* 4th ed. New York: Free Press.

Bayer. 2016. "Our Mission; Bayer; Science for a Better Life." Accessed June 8. www.bayer.com/en/mission---values.aspx.

Copeland, M. K. 2014. "The Emerging Significance of Values Based Leadership: A Literature Review." *International Journal of Leadership Studies* 8 (2): 105–35.

Dye, C. F., and B. D. Lee. 2016. *The Healthcare Leader's Guide to Actions, Awareness, and Perception*, 3rd ed. Chicago: Health Administration Press.

Forrestal, E. J., and L. W. Cellucci. 2016. *Ethics and Professionalism for Healthcare Managers*. Chicago: Health Administration Press.

Frost, R. 2016. "The Road Not Taken." Poetry Foundation. Accessed June 17. www.poetryfoundation.org/resources/learning/core-poems/detail/44272.

George, B. 2004. *Authentic Leadership: Rediscovering the Secrets to Creating Lasting Value*. New York: John Wiley & Sons.

Hughes, R. L., R. C. Ginnett, and G. J. Curphy. 2015. *Leadership: Enhancing the Lessons of Experience*, 8th ed. Burr Ridge, IL: McGraw-Hill Education.

Kraemer, H. M. J. Jr. 2011. *From Values to Action: The Four Principles of Values-Based Leadership*. San Francisco: Jossey-Bass.

Kreitner, R., and A. Kinicki. 2012. *Organizational Behavior*, 10th ed. Burr Ridge, IL: McGraw-Hill Education.

Muscat, E., and M. Whitty. 2009. "Social Entrepreneurship: Values-Based Leadership to Transform Business Education and Society." *Business Renaissance Quarterly* 4 (1): 31–44.

Northouse, P. G. 2016. *Leadership: Theory and Practice*, 7th ed. Los Angeles: SAGE Publications.

Pavlina, S. 2004. "List of Values." StevePavlina.com. Published November 29. www.stevepavlina.com/articles/list-of-values.htm.

Roberts, W. 1989. *Leadership Secrets of Attila the Hun*. New York: Warner Books.

Sarros, J. C., and J. C. Santora. 2001. "Leadership and Values: A Cross-Cultural Study." *Leadership and Organization Development Journal* 22 (5): 243–48.

SUGGESTED READINGS

Alexander, C., D. Campbell, J. Leiferman, G. Mabey, S. Marken, C. Myers, A. Pengra, T. Reyburn-Orne, T. S. Sundem, and C. Zwingman-Bagley. 2003. "Quality Improvement Processes in Growing a Service Line." *Nursing Administration Quarterly* 27 (4): 297–306.

Brown, M. E., and L. K. Treviño. 2006. "Socialized Charismatic Leadership, Values Congruence, and Deviance in Work Groups." *Journal of Applied Psychology* 91 (4): 954–62.

Carmeli, A., and M. Y. Halevi. 2009. "How Top Management Team Behavioral Integration and Behavioral Complexity Enable Organizational Ambidexterity: The Moderating Role of Contextual Ambidexterity." *Leadership Quarterly* 20 (2): 207–18.

Clark, L. 2008. "Clinical Leadership: Values, Beliefs and Vision." *Nursing Management* 15 (7): 30–35.

Dye, C. F., and A. N. Garman. 2015. *Exceptional Leadership: 16 Critical Competencies for Healthcare Leaders*, 2nd ed. Chicago: Health Administration Press.

Garman, A. N., and M. Johnson. 2006. "Leadership Competencies: An Introduction." *Journal of Healthcare Management* 51 (1): 13–17.

Hughes, R. L., R. C. Ginnett, and G. J. Curphy. 2015. *Leadership: Enhancing the Lessons of Experience*, 8th ed. Burr Ridge, IL: McGraw-Hill Education.

Karp, T., and T. I. Tveteraas Helgø. 2009. "Reality Revisited: Leading People in Chaotic Change." *Journal of Management Development* 28 (2): 81–93.

Miles, R. E. 2007. "Innovation and Leadership Values." *California Management Review* 50 (1): 192–201.

Reave, L. 2005. "Spiritual Values and Practices Related to Leadership Effectiveness." *Leadership Quarterly* 16 (5): 655–87.

Souba, W. W., and D. V. Day. 2006. "Leadership Values in Academic Medicine." *Academic Medicine: Journal of the Association of American Medical Colleges* 81 (1): 20–26.

Souba, W. W., D. Mauger, and D. V. Day. 2007. "Does Agreement on Institutional Values and Leadership Issues Between Deans and Surgery Chairs Predict Their Institutions' Performance?" *Academic Medicine: Journal of the Association of American Medical Colleges* 82 (3): 272–80.

Stanley, D. 2008. "Congruent Leadership: Values in Action." *Journal of Nursing Management* 16 (5): 519–24.

Yukl, G. 2010. *Leadership in Organizations*, 7th ed. Upper Saddle River, NJ: Prentice Hall.

CHAPTER 5

The Senior Leader Challenge

*Health care delivery is arguably
the most complex industry in existence.*

—John Glaser (2013)

THE CHALLENGES IN healthcare have been about the same for many years, centering on finance and quality. However, some of these issues have become more critical and new ones have surfaced, as mentioned in chapter 1. Following are specific challenges that senior leadership teams have encountered in the past few years:

- Legislative change—the Affordable Care Act, perhaps the most substantive law since Medicare and Medicaid
- New risk model—move toward pay for value, clinical integration, population health management, accountable care organizations
- Physicians—shortages, recruitment, retention, engagement, generational changes
- Care outside the acute care facility—the need to control, or at least partially manage, non-post-acute care
- Improving outcomes, readmission prevention, increased emphasis on patient quality and safety
- Bigger entities—insurance company mergers, collaboratives

- Patients and families—their involvement within a consumer-driven market and retail healthcare
- Information technology (IT) implementation—massive systems, including the 10th edition of International Statistical Classification of Diseases and Related Health Problems

Exhibit 5.1 describes the four-pronged challenges facing the field. This chapter gives voice to leaders' main concerns—be they internal or external to their organizations and the field. The intent here is to raise awareness of the fact that values-driven leaders have an advantage over these seemingly insurmountable challenges.

ORGANIZATIONAL FACTORS

Now more than ever, senior leaders need to depend on their strong values to effectively lead their hospitals and health systems. Chaos

Exhibit 5.1 The Four-Pronged Challenge

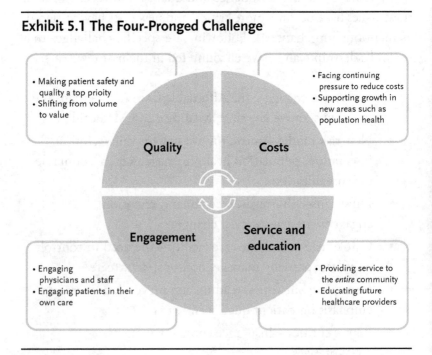

- Making patient safety and quality a top prioity
- Shifting from volume to value

Quality

- Facing continuing pressure to reduce costs
- Supporting growth in new areas such as population health

Costs

Engagement

- Engaging physicians and staff
- Engaging patients in their own care

Service and education

- Providing service to the *entire* community
- Educating future healthcare providers

sometimes arises in part because leaders fail to anticipate, work through, and rise above the inevitable changes in the field. To be fair, however, organizational factors do exist that can impede leaders' performance and can exacerbate the effects of current challenges. These factors are described in this section.

Complex Organizational Structure

Mergers, acquisitions, alliances, affiliations, coalitions, federations, and other types of partnerships reinvented how healthcare services are delivered, paid for, and measured. This redesign created the need for more managers to oversee the quality and flow of even more services. Ultimately, a vast structural maze of managers with various titles emerged. Moreover, the growth of collaboratives has introduced an innovative—but not fully developed—organizational structure.

Many hospitals have become health systems, and to flourish or at least survive in a competitive market, they have created multiple business lines and adopted new approaches. Often, this expansion has created a schism between leaders who are involved in only external transactions (e.g., physician practice acquisitions, alliances, new business lines) and those who oversee day-to-day operations.

Rapid growth has also diversified the composition and enlarged the size of the typical senior leadership team. As a result, the personal and professional camaraderie that used to bind leaders is almost extinct, and the meetings have become too large for intimate and goal-driven interaction. Some teams convene as many as 20 to 30 people. Both research and common sense prove that a team this large cannot be effective. De Rond (2012) writes that "people tend to prefer teams of four or, at most, five members. Anything lower than four was felt to be too small to be effective, whereas teams larger than five became ineffective." And Hackman (Coutu 2009) states that "as a team gets bigger, the number of links that need to be managed among members goes up at an accelerating, almost exponential rate. It's managing the links between members that gets teams into trouble. My rule of thumb is no double digits."

A senior leadership team with more than 20 individuals is not at all unusual today. One executive laments that "our leadership team meets for longer periods of time and wastes more time than ever before." Some teams have become orchestrated show-and-tell sessions where the primary goal seems to be for each leader to showcase her great accomplishments. Rarely can teams of a large size engage in any true problem solving. Readers may want to ponder the *Bezos rule* (named after Amazon.com founder Jeff Bezos): Teams must be small enough to feed with only two pizzas (Brandt 2011).

Haphazard Executive Search Process

Little preparation or forethought is given to the executive hiring process; organizations usually just jump in to start recruitment. Although employers are clear on their intentions to search extensively and select the best candidate, they are vague on the actual execution of this plan. This type of hiring may also be classified as *start and stop*, whereby the organization moves quickly to advertise the vacancy or contracts with a search firm, then pauses the process for an indefinite period, and then slowly reenters it before getting back on track. Here, the message seems to be that the employer has bigger priorities, forcing it to delay the recruitment process.

Poor preparation causes executive hiring decisions to be made too subjectively or on gut-feeling, not based on the organization's true needs or the position's expectations and qualifications. With gut-feeling hiring, many executive search processes become an endurance test for those involved, focusing almost exclusively on interpersonal style and fit. Sometimes the unfortunate result is the selection of a leader who has inadequate leadership competencies (see chapter 2) and knowledge of healthcare.

Moreover, with increasing leadership shortages, many organizations have realized that searching for candidates from outside the organization is no longer a viable option. More healthcare systems are devoting substantial resources to in-house leadership development programs. This trend is even more true of physician leadership, where the external supply is greatly limited and the risks involved in a hiring mistake are astronomical.

Litigious Environment

Some challenges faced by leaders today are new. Because these leaders have had no prior knowledge of or experience with the matters at hand, their decisions are often based on best guesses—a risky and potentially fatal move.

The legal ramifications of some of these issues further complicate decision-making processes. Recent challenges such as developing telehealth, protecting or securing the voluminous personal data compiled in IT systems, and instituting better corporate governance policies have compounded the complexity of legal issues in healthcare. With the continued growth of systems and consolidations, antitrust considerations become important. One CEO remarks that the "mission too often takes the back seat to legal maneuvering."

As providers, payers, governments, and other stakeholders strive to deliver effective, efficient, and equitable care, they do so in an ecosystem that is undergoing a dramatic and fundamental shift in business, clinical, and operating models. This shift is being fueled by aging and growing populations; the proliferation of chronic diseases; heightened focus on care quality and value; evolving financial and quality regulations; informed and empowered consumers; and innovative treatments and technologies—all of which are leading to rising costs and an increase in spending levels for care provision, infrastructure improvements, and technology innovations.

—Deloitte (2016)

Fast Pace of Change

The traditional mind-set in healthcare is to follow predictable, tried processes; therefore, many of its leaders are reluctant to adopt innovative or even alternative strategies or methods of operation. The proliferation of information on the Internet and the fast speed at

> The cacophony of models ranging from strictly fee for service to pay for performance, care management/patient-centered medical home, bundled payment, shared savings/ACO, full or partial risk/capitation and beyond will continue to add administrative, strategic, operational, and financial complexity to most organizations. Trying to make sense of this blend of payment structures from both a financial and a care model perspective will cause continued confusion before the fog clears.
>
> —Laura Jacobs (2016)

which this information can be accessed encourage leaders to change with the times and make fast decisions. In fact, leaders who are reluctant to take part in a modern, technological world are seen as a liability because they fail to anticipate and thus capitalize on innovation and other advances. On the other hand, leaders who are advocates and first adopters of new technology are said to be informed, headed in the right direction, and even ahead of the competition.

Those characterizations may be right. However, there is a casualty in this fast-moving trend: The quality of the decisions suffers because leaders do not have enough time to consult with each other or to reflect on the implications of their decisions. A CEO from the Midwest admits that her board is often frustrated with the number and speed of significant decisions that her team has to make without thoughtful deliberation.

Decision making without proper analysis is prevalent in any industry; it is a product of the rapidly transforming world, with or without the Internet, mobile devices, and other technology-based media. A leader's strong values can help when both time and information are limited but demands are endless.

Lack of Time

Lack of time (specifically, the constant pressure to produce or decide in a limited time) has resulted in burnout and stress.

In addition, lack of time has led to the following:

- *Communication problems.* Because the meeting agenda is filled with so many pressing issues, not all members of the leadership team can convey their thoughts. Even those who have the opportunity to do so cannot properly elaborate on their ideas. On the other hand, some leaders may counter that so much time is spent on meeting minutiae that less time is appropriated for actual strategy evaluation.

- *Less interaction among leaders.* Frontline managers spend more time working together than do senior leaders. Many executive team members come together only occasionally and thus are less familiar and friendly with each other. At this level, personal and professional conflicts tend to be more common and can be more volatile. Competitive members use insider knowledge to intimidate and subdue opposing members. Knowledge is frequently withheld.

- *Reliance on e-mail.* Time-strapped leaders share information and consult about decisions through e-mail. While this method is more efficient than a phone call, it prevents the proper airing out of issues and causes the input of stakeholders who are not privy to the e-mail sequence to be overlooked.

Lack of Shared Vision

Goals are achievable only when everyone on the team is deeply committed to them. Unfortunately, some executive team members move in the opposite direction from the rest of the team, have self-serving agendas, and possess little personal or professional compatibility with colleagues. While some leaders focus on external business development activities, others commit to managing acute care outcomes. Senior-level goals such as improving health system performance or enhancing quality and patient safety are broader and more abstract than the goals set by middle management teams. The threat of losing their jobs, which is always a possibility, especially in a financially difficult time, can turn some leaders into fierce competitors and create a negative political landscape.

CONCLUSION

One of the most important characteristics of strong leaders is the ability to objectively analyze their performance and their impact on the organization. This must be done with a full realization of the challenge factors described in this chapter. Highly effective leaders must keep a keen eye on the external factors affecting their organizations while at the same time assessing and measuring their own personal leadership performance. Part IV of this book provides various assessment tools. Consider the concepts in this chapter and apply them to your organization.

Self-Evaluation Questions

❏ How influential is the senior leadership team in my organization?

❏ Does the frequent turnover among senior leaders create a serious, negative effect on the team's effectiveness? Why?

❏ What is my organization doing to increase the number of and quality of physician leaders?

Exercises

Exercise 5.1

Question: Which group has the greater ability to change an organization—senior leaders or middle managers?

Viewpoint: Senior leaders have far more impact and ability to change an organization for several reasons. First, they create and interpret organizational policies. Second, they assess the environment and develop strategy. Third, they control the budget and make the ultimate decisions regarding executive hires. Fourth, they have better insight into environmental trends than do middle managers. Last, their span of control is greater, and they work closely with the board.

Do you agree with this viewpoint? Why? Why not? What points do you think are untrue of today's senior leaders?

Exercise 5.2

The layers of hierarchy between a senior leader and a middle manager continue to peel off in many industries, including healthcare. Using information gleaned from the Internet, contrast the role and activities of a senior leader with those of a middle manager. If possible, interview a senior leader and a middle manager.

Exercise 5.2 Questions

1. What are the typical responsibilities of a senior leader?

2. What are the typical responsibilities of a middle manager?

3. How is a senior leader rewarded and recognized? How do these acknowledgments differ from those received by a middle manager?

Suggested Readings for Exercise 5.2

- Henri Fayol's span of control theory may be found in any organizational behavior textbook. An excellent summary can be found at www.stybelpeabody.com/newsite/pdf/ceotime.pdf.

- Amy McCutcheon and Ruth Anne Campbell's "Leadership, Span of Control, Turnover, Staff and

(continued)

(continued from previous page)

Patient Satisfaction." This article discusses the relationships among span of control, employee turnover, and patient satisfaction. See http://stti.confex.com/stti/inrc16/techprogram/paper_23430.htm.

REFERENCES

Brandt, R. L. 2011. "Birth of a Salesman." *Wall Street Journal*. Published October 15. www.wsj.com/articles/SB10001424052970 20391430457662710299683120.

Coutu, D. 2009. "Why Teams Don't Work." Interview of J. Richard Hackman, the Edgar Pierce Professor of Social and Organizational Psychology at Harvard University. *Harvard Business Review*. Published May. https://hbr.org/2009/05/why-teams-dont-work.

Deloitte. 2016. *2016 Global Health Care Outlook: Battling Costs While Improving Care*. Accessed January 31. www2.deloitte.com/content/dam/Deloitte/global/Documents/Life-Sciences-Health-Care/gx-lshc-2016-health-care-outlook.pdf.

de Rond, M. 2012. "Why Less Is More in Teams." *Harvard Business Review*. Published August 6. https://hbr.org/2012/08/why-less-is-more-in-teams/.

Glaser, J. 2013. "Managing Complexity with Health Care Information Technology." *H&HN Daily*. Published October 8. www.hhnmag.com/articles/6094-managing-complexity-with-health-care-information-technology.

Jacobs, L. 2016. "Looking Ahead in 2016: Top 10 Trends in Health Care." *H&HN Daily*. Published January 5. www.hhnmag.com/articles/6800-looking-ahead-in---top---trends-in-health-care.

PART II

PERSONAL VALUES

CHAPTER 6

Respect as the
Foundation of Leadership

*When people respect you only because of your
authority, they will give you the minimum effort.*

—Jim Whitehurst (2015)

JOHN GEORGE, A system CEO, and Julia Garrison, a senior
vice president, were overheard discussing the beginning of
the era of clinical integration and pay for value:

JULIA. John, healthcare seems to have greatly changed since
you first entered it 25 years ago. The field and its workers
are not as respected today. Would you agree?

JOHN. When I entered healthcare, many of us saw healthcare
management as a calling. We wanted to serve people, to
make a difference. I think now too many people go into it
as just another career.

JULIA. I'm not sure I agree. Most of us new administrators
are still service oriented. The problem is that healthcare

leaders have been viewed as villains, even though we do a lot, directly and indirectly, to improve the health and lives of our patients and our workers. Don't you think the old days of the command-and-control healthcare CEOs may have something to do with this negative public perception? I think we could make some changes in our leadership's attitudes that would have a profound impact on our patients, physicians, and employees.

JOHN. Perhaps you're right, although I wouldn't say autocratic leaders are now a relic of the past. Unfortunately, they still exist, and they certainly harm the reputation of all healthcare administrators. I think, though, that the real requirement today is to have a deep and profound respect for workers and the care and services they provide.

Here is my challenge to you: Talk with your colleagues, do some research, and make a recommendation about how to effect a sea change in management. We'll discuss your findings, and we'll see how we can implement changes in our own backyard, so to speak.

RESPECT IS THE value that multiplies the desire of both the leader and follower to work harder and deliver consistently excellent performance.

Leadership has traditionally been perceived as a prestigious position filled by influential people whose main role is to give orders and impose inflexible rules. This misconception may not be as prevalent now because more leaders have become aware that autocratic management begets only few and uneasy followers. Society frequently rejects selfish leadership. This type of behavior repeatedly leads to entitlement, greed, and other feelings of privilege, as has been frequently reported in the media in the

> Leaders who respect others also allow them to be themselves, with creative wants and desires. They approach other people with a sense of their unconditional worth and valuable individual differences.
>
> —Peter G. Northouse (2016)

past decade. As a result, many Americans distrust and are cynical about the C-suite—not just in healthcare but in all industries.

Respect for self and others is the nucleus of all activities, especially in management. It is a value that enables leaders to restrain ego, admit mistakes, pay attention, care about and honor others, keep an open mind, give credit or compliments, and ask for help or insight. Leaders must return to this basic value to regain trust and amplify their effectiveness. Although the task is daunting, the undertaking is worthwhile.

For many years now, I have spoken and written about the protocols of leadership. These protocols are the often unwritten behavioral rules society and organizations expect from their leaders. These generally accepted standards of behavior cannot possibly cover all situations faced by leaders, but they share a common element: respect.

This chapter makes a distinction between self-esteem and self-centeredness, two opposing forces in management style. While self-esteem boosts the persuasiveness of a leader, self-centeredness undermines it altogether. In addition, the chapter also suggests several approaches for showing and gaining respect (see exhibit 6.1).

SELF-ESTEEM VERSUS SELF-CENTEREDNESS

Self-esteem is an individual's respect for her own convictions, actions, imperfections, and abilities. Without self-esteem, a person is not

---

Exhibit 6.1 How to Show Respect for Others

1. Give compliments, be courteous, and demonstrate good manners and pleasant deportment to show that you appreciate and honor the efforts that others bring to the organization.

2. Learn the strength of collective action through the cooperative work of teams.

3. Ask and listen to what others value, need, and expect.

4. Participate in others' activities to show you care about their interests.

---

mentally healthy; does not function well under pressure; cannot accept or give compliments and criticism; and tends to be egotistical, controlling, and in constant need of affirmation.

Self-centeredness, on the other hand, is an individual's overly favorable sense of his own abilities, views, decisions, and needs. A self-centered person is arrogant, insecure (yet feels superior), and a nuisance (if not harmful) in any social or professional setting.

Leaders who have low self-esteem but are highly self-centered

- do not respect or trust others;
- alienate others with a domineering attitude;
- are exasperating because they seek and demand so much approval;
- cause unnecessary work and waste time; and
- engender disloyalty, stress, and fear.

Exhibit 6.2 contrasts self-esteem with self-centeredness.

Exhibit 6.2 Self-Esteem Versus Self-Centeredness

Self-Esteem		Self-Centeredness
Respects self	vs.	Has overly favorable concept of self
Accepts and gives compliments and criticism gracefully	vs.	Demands constant approval while being unduly critical
Collaborates and cooperates with others	vs.	Alienates others with an arrogant approach
Stays efficient by relying on colleagues for aid	vs.	Doubts others, creating unnecessary work
Cultivates an inclusive, team-oriented atmosphere	vs.	Fosters disloyalty and suspicion in the workplace

THE CONCEPT IN PRACTICE

Following are some ways a leader can show respect in various facets of her position.

Become a Collaborator

Collaboration is a partnership among people who have shared goals but distinct strategies or priorities. The reasons for collaboration are varied and include the desire to expedite achievement of results; combine expertise, experience, and resources; minimize or prevent mistakes and waste in effort, time, and money; and produce a better product.

Leaders who become good collaborators learn to

- hold judgment until all the variables and others' opinions have been presented;
- listen actively;
- reflect before responding; and
- ask questions to understand, not to cast doubt.

Exhibit 6.3 is a basic guide to effective collaboration.

Senior leaders must push other executives to seek collaborations with those in lower-level positions. Why is this necessary? Because collaboration is about the equal exchange of ideas, not a privileged activity of those at the top of the organizational hierarchy. An inter-office collaboration that includes multilevel partners is a sign that leaders respect the insights and contributions of all employees.

Be Aware of Others' Definition of Respect

Respect means different things to different people. For example, Person A may perceive respect when he is asked for his opinion,

Exhibit 6.3 Key Requirements of Effective Collaboration

Common desired outcome. The collaboration must offer a reciprocal benefit to all partners or participants. The stakeholders must believe that they are getting something good in return for their efforts and that the end product improves the current situation.

Shared responsibility. The driving force of a true collaboration is shared responsibility—from decision making to implementation to monitoring and assessment. All members of the partnership, not just its leaders, must be able to voice their concerns, opinions, and questions. Consensus must be reached at all times. Responsibility for failure or negative consequences must also be shared by all involved.

Support. In a collaborative situation, parties to the process support each other's right to express ideas and suggestions. When a decision is made to move forward, all stakeholders support the conclusion.

Clear objective. The group must have a clear understanding of the collaboration's purpose or goal.

Trust. Trust is built when all partners commit to being transparent and sharing information. A willingness to admit mistakes also helps in this regard.

Open communication. Suspending judgment, not assigning blame, actively listening, being interested and inquisitive, and checking in or following up promote open communication among collaborators.

Celebration. Gains and accomplishments must be celebrated. Doing so encourages participants.

---

while Person B may feel respected if she is empowered to make an important decision.

For many people, the level of respect they give, get, or demand depends on superficial attributes such as job title. Unfortunately, respect for those who clean the facilities, for example, seems nonexistent in many industries. Likewise, professors and students alike may not show as much respect for their university's security personnel or cafeteria staff. In clinical practice, physicians are traditionally more respected than are nurses or allied health profession-als. In management, executives garner more respect than do receptionists and other frontline employees.

A good leader understands these dynamics and recognizes everyone's human dignity and basic need for respect. When asked how he shows respect, a successful CEO says, "I hire the very best people I can find, and then I show them the respect they are due by staying out of their way and letting them do their jobs." Another high-performing CEO reveals, "All of my executive team members think and act like each is my COO [chief operations officer]— and most important, they make most of their deci-sions without my involvement." These two quotes exemplify how leaders can show respect by empowering their staff.

> Being in a position to exercise power over other people . . . may be satisfying for a little while, but never in the long run. Ultimately it leaves you lonely. You command, and you receive fear and obedience in return, and what emotionally healthy person can live on a diet of fear and obedience?
>
> —Harold S. Kushner (1986)

Establish a Feedback System

The best feedback systems are those that provide constant, unfiltered, direct feedback and, when necessary, criticism. Feedback should be given on an ongoing basis and should be informal. The recipient of the feedback should be given an opportunity to respond, ask ques-tions, or simply confirm his understanding.

In the book *Giving and Receiving Performance Feedback*, author Peter Garber (2004) indicates that in most organizations, it has become increasingly rare that true open dialogue occurs in tradi-tional performance evaluation sessions. Executives' interactions are more often than not held in the C-suite, a setting that can intimidate most people. The fact that the leaders giving the evaluation have the power to hire and fire adds to the tension. As a result of these trappings, leaders may be less skilled at evaluating their direct reports and vice versa (Garman and Dye 2009).

> It is difficult to imagine how work group or team performance could improve without feedback.
>
> —Richard L. Hughes, Robert C. Ginnett, and Gordon J. Curphy (2015)

Seeking and accepting feedback is a sign of respect, communicating that others' opinions are valued. When leaders interact with staff regularly, they appear accessible and are better informed.

Be Genuine

Genuineness is referred to as *authentic presence*. It can be conveyed by being visibly involved in organizational activities and showing a vested interest in others' work without being intrusive and pretentious. The unspoken message here is that "we are in this together." Forman (2010, 4) states, "We need to listen with what has been called the 'third ear.' This requires an open mind that embraces discovery and welcomes possibilities. To do this, we must temporarily set aside what we think or know and listen carefully."

Many CEOs practice management by walking around (MBWA), a popular strategy among leaders. MBWA's primary purpose is to witness the effectiveness or ineffectiveness of various services and, by extension, those who perform the work. Although MBWA provides great insight and breeds familiarity, it should be carefully managed to ensure that employees believe the approach is sincere.

In Catholic hospitals, nuns (many of them top administrators) traditionally were known to be extraordinary influencers because they were frequently visible and consistently approachable. Physicians tend to gravitate toward physician leaders who

> This dialogue from the classic tale *The Velveteen Rabbit* (Williams 1922, 3–4) serves as a reminder of how everyone can develop an authentic presence.
>
> "What is REAL?" asked the Rabbit one day. . . . "Does it mean having things that buzz inside you and a stick-out handle?"
>
> "Real isn't how you are made," said the Skin Horse. "It's a thing that happens to you. . . ."
>
> "Does it hurt?" asked the Rabbit.
>
> "Sometimes," said the Skin Horse, for he was always truthful. "When you are Real you don't mind being hurt."
>
> "Does it happen all at once, like being wound up," he asked, "or bit by bit?"
>
> "It doesn't happen all at once," said the Skin Horse. "You become. It takes a long time. That's why it doesn't often happen to people who break easily, or have sharp edges, or who have to be carefully kept. . . . Once you are Real you can't be ugly, except to people who don't understand."

are frequently seen in clinical areas and believe such leaders can better represent their needs, understand their concerns, and defend their demands. This tendency is even more true for the physician leaders who maintain some amount of clinical practice.

Give Credit and Acknowledge Accomplishments

The mark of a great leader is his ability to step back from the spotlight and publicly recognize someone else's excellent performance. This simple acknowledgment is one of the most powerful motivators, much quieter than a standing ovation but more valuable than money.

Offer Help or Coaching

Many leaders study coaching to enhance their abilities to evaluate, constructively criticize, and assist their staff's performance. By helping staff develop, the leader is saying, "I admire and respect your work so much that I want to invest in your growth and accomplishments."

Be Self-Aware

Leaders must be able to look inward to discover their strengths, weaknesses, goals, and impetus. Creativity often springs from being self-aware. In *Exceptional Leadership*, well-cultivated self-awareness is one of the four key cornerstones of superb leadership (Dye and Garman 2015). This approach requires strong feedback mechanisms as well as a willingness to consider with an open mind the input received.

> Résumé virtues are what we write about ourselves to measure up to the world's expectations. Eulogy virtues are what others say about us at our funeral: what kind of person we were and how we cared for others.
>
> —Bill George (2016)

Take Responsibility for Mistakes and Apologize

This approach is often the most overlooked way of showing respect. Many leaders fail to realize that by simply owning up to their mistakes and apologizing, they are loudly proclaiming that they are penetrable, they are vincible, and they are human—hence, on the same level as others. What others hear when leaders say "I made a mistake and I'm sorry" is "I respect you, so I will not pretend or make you believe that what happened was your responsibility."

Learn the Principle of Affirmation

The word *affirm* comes from an ancient legal principle: The higher court must approve the decision of the lower court. In hospitals and health systems, leaders function as the higher court that affirms the work and contributions of their employees (the lower court). This principle serves as a powerful, positive message and a great motivator for better performance.

Positive affirmations are statements and behaviors that build others up and boost their confidence and sense of well-being. They serve to minimize the many negative distractions that occur in the workplace. The advice that leaders give in the workplace and the atmosphere created by leaders in an organization help to shape the attitude that others in that organization have.

Show Appreciation

A note of congratulations, appreciation, or gratitude has always been a staple of good camaraderie. Many leaders still make time to handwrite notes, but this practice has declined as e-mails, phone calls, video conferences or chats, and even texts have become more common for their convenience and speed. Whatever the means of delivery, the idea is the same: A small token makes a big impression.

Show Enthusiasm

Some leaders may think that showing enthusiasm about an endeavor is inappropriate, unprofessional, or even silly. However, it has a positive effect on followers. Enthusiasm can energize people and boost loyalty to the undertaking.

Showing enthusiasm and support for the mission of the organization is also important because the rank and file models the behavior of its leaders. Employees can become cynical if they only hear but do not see their leaders' support of the mission.

Enthusiasm may also be expressed through attending or participating in employee events. Failure to make an appearance or embrace these events can drive a wedge between the C-suite and the front line, perpetuating the perception that senior leaders are only interested in activities that revolve around the power structure. As one executive's flippant remark expresses, "I really see no sense in serving hot dogs at the employee picnic. Let others handle that, and I'll handle my job."

CONCLUSION

Respect may be commonsense knowledge to some leaders. However, the concept is surprisingly novel to many others. Admittedly, showing respect is hard to master, and convincing people to try it is even harder, especially in today's healthcare workplace already overwhelmed with too many "must dos." But giving respect is not a temporary fix or trend; it is a fundamental value in all aspects of life.

Cases and Exercise

Case 6.1

Roberto Santiago has been CEO of St. James for the past three years, hired for his strategic visioning acumen. He spends his time in meetings with board members, community leaders, and physicians. Recently, he led a successful strategic planning retreat, garnering him strong support from the board and medical staff.

Roberto has put Jane Robbins, the chief operations officer, in charge of running St. James's daily operations. Jane oversees the vice presidents and attends all staff meetings. During a monthly housekeeping meeting, Jane fielded questions from the housekeeping staff. One asked, "We never see Mr. Santiago. Does he not care what happens to us?"

How would you answer this question if you were Jane?

Case 6.2

Courtney Sample is the new hard-charging, tough-as-nails CEO of a system hospital. She is well known for delivering great results, but sometimes at the expense of many. Previously, she executed a multiyear, multimillion-dollar turnaround of a bankrupt hospital, replacing the entire senior leadership team in the process.

Six months into her position, Courtney is frustrated. She has not been able to finish a single project, and morale among her senior leadership team is at an all-time low. Many of the employees and physicians are unfamiliar with her, and those who know her avoid eye contact. She schedules an appointment with her longtime personal coach, Will Cheng, to seek his guidance. Will spends a day talking with Courtney's staff and then meets her over dinner.

WILL. You intimidate your staff. They didn't even want to talk to me. They think you view them like tools, just there to get the job done.

COURTNEY. Isn't that what we all are anyway? Tools to get the job done?

Case 6.2 Questions

1. How can showing respect help Courtney out of this scenario? What can Will do and say to correct Courtney's misguided attitude?

2. How is the concept of respect a constant in all leadership settings? Consider the leader who states, "Sometimes, I want my followers to fear me." Is this dynamic ever appropriate?

Exercise 6.1

Review one of the following academic articles and describe its findings on the role of respect in leadership.

Clarke, N. 2011. "An Integrated Conceptual Model of Respect in Leadership." *Leadership Quarterly* 22 (2): 316–27.

(continued)

(continued from previous page)

Ulrich, B. T., P. I. Buerhaus, K. Donelan, L. Norman, and R. Dittus. 2005. "How RNs View the Work Environment: Results of a National Survey of Registered Nurses." *Journal of Nursing Administration* 35 (9): 389–96.

REFERENCES

Dye, C. F., and A. N. Garman. 2015. *Exceptional Leadership: 16 Critical Competencies for Healthcare Leaders*, 2nd ed. Chicago: Health Administration Press.

Forman, H. 2010. *Nursing Leadership for Patient-Centered Care: Authenticity, Presence, Intuition, Expertise.* New York: Springer Publishing Company.

Garber, P. R. 2004. *Giving and Receiving Performance Feedback.* Amherst, MA: HRD Press.

Garman, A. N., and C. F. Dye. 2009. *The Healthcare C-Suite: Leadership Development at the Top.* Chicago: Health Administration Press.

George, B. 2016. "What's Your Life Goal? Success or Significance?" Published April 27. www.billgeorge.org/page/fortune-whats-your-life-goal-success-or-significance.

Hughes, R. L., R. C. Ginnett, and G. J. Curphy. 2015. *Leadership: Enhancing the Lessons of Experience*, 8th ed. Burr Ridge, IL: McGraw-Hill Education.

Kushner, H. S. 1986. *When All You've Ever Wanted Isn't Enough: The Search for a Life That Matters.* New York: Simon and Schuster.

Northouse, P. G. 2016. *Leadership: Theory and Practice*, 7th ed. Los Angeles: SAGE Publications.

Whitehurst, J. 2015. *The Open Organization: Igniting Passion and Performance*. Boston: Harvard Business Review Press.

Williams, M. 1922. *The Velveteen Rabbit, or How Toys Become Real*. London: Heinemann.

SUGGESTED READINGS

Day, D. V., J. W. Fleenor, L. E. Atwater, R. E. Sturm, and R. A. McKee. 2014. "Advances in Leader and Leadership Development: A Review of 25 Years of Research and Theory." *Leadership Quarterly* 25 (1): 63–82.

Ghutke, S., R. Jaiswal, and A. Thakur. 2014. "Case Analysis of 360 Degree Feedback." *International Journal of Advanced Research in Education, Technology and Management* 2 (3): 202–6.

CHAPTER 7

Ethics and Integrity

*Leaders with integrity inspire confidence
in others because they can be trusted to do
what they say they are going to do.*

—Peter G. Northouse (2016)

IN A POPULAR graduate health administration course, the professor turns to the topic of ethics: "How important is ethics in healthcare leadership? And how do we determine that someone is truly ethical?"

STUDENT A. First, you have to define what a leader is supposed to do. Then, you can determine the ethics from there.

STUDENT B. It's all about the end result. Outcomes are important in healthcare; that's what we are here to do—help make positive changes for people.

STUDENT C. I have a problem with the idea that something is ethical just because it benefits a great number of people. That shortchanges the role that values need to play in leadership. What about the minority number who are inevitably disadvantaged by the change? Don't they count? What about the leader who ignored her moral compass just so she could provide for the many?

STUDENT D. But I think we're missing the core of the matter—frankly, if leaders don't have high integrity and ethics, they're not effective.

PROFESSOR. Excellent responses! There are no easy answers in ethics, which is why it's important to have discussions about these issues.

AS ARE OTHER leadership values, ethics and integrity are interrelated. Ethics is a person's moral scope, and integrity is the person's capacity for staying within that moral scope. The general concept of both values is comprehensible, but their true meaning is elusive.

This chapter explores the tandem nature of ethics and integrity. It provides a guide for leaders on how to practice ethical behavior within the constructs of daily operation. While the vignette presents both a macro view and a micro view of ethics, this chapter focuses on leaders' daily activities.

DEFINING INTEGRITY

Practically all leaders believe they possess high integrity. However, when asked to name other leaders who have integrity, many demur by saying, "Integrity is hard to define." Why the contradiction? Three reasons are plausible.

> Leaders who do not behave ethically do not demonstrate true leadership.
>
> —J. M. Burns (1978)

First, many definitions for integrity exist, but none is universal. According to the *Merriam Webster's Collegiate Dictionary*, Eleventh Edition, integrity is "the quality or state of being complete or undivided." To some people, the word could mean absolute honesty, while to others, it is a high degree of genuineness. My definition is that it is the quality that allows a person to differentiate right from wrong. Northouse (2016, 27), meanwhile, defines it this way: "Basically, integrity makes a leader believable and worthy of our trust." Each definition almost always reflects a person's sensibility (e.g., moral compass, bias, expectation). Thus, applying it to others can be a difficult proposition.

Second, our perception of integrity varies from one situation to the next. Everyone has his own concept of right and wrong, but we all stray occasionally from our own standards. For example, if Leader A, who is regularly lauded for her good ethical judgment, occasionally uses the organization's copy machine to copy personal paperwork or uses the company's computer to surf the Internet on her lunch hour, is she being unethical? Although Leader A's sensibility informs her that these actions are inappropriate, she continues because she does not deem them harmful to the organization. This scenario is an example of *ethical relativism* or contingency leadership. It provokes leaders into considering their own ethical anchors before facing complex situations.

Third, although difficult to define, integrity still ranks at or near the top of all lists of required leadership traits. Palanski and Yammarino (2007, 171) state that the "study of integrity, however, suffers from three significant problems: too many definitions, too little theory, and too few rigorous empirical studies." (This is the same argument I made in chapter 3 about popular leadership literature.) Nevertheless, many leadership books provide ample space for discussing integrity.

> When you clarify the principles that will govern your life and the ends that you will seek, you give purpose to your daily decisions. A personal creed gives you a point of reference for navigating the sometimes-stormy seas of organizational life. Without such a set of beliefs, your life has no rudder, and you are easily blown about by the winds of fashion. A credo that resolves competing beliefs also leads to personal integrity.
>
> —James M. Kouzes and Barry Z. Posner (2012)

THE CONCEPT IN PRACTICE

The ethical decisions of leaders, especially senior executives, are observed more closely—and are likely more scrutinized—than any other decisions they make. An ethical dilemma bears significant personal and professional risk because its resolution often compels a leader to reveal her private opinions. How can leaders lessen this risk but still handle these ethical challenges? The following approaches serve as a guide.

Adopt an Organizational Code of Ethics

An organizational code of ethics defines appropriate and inappropriate conduct in the workplace and identifies conduct that falls between those poles. It protects the organization from legal entanglement and employees from harassment and unfair treatment. Leaders should be enlisted to support the code and should educate themselves and others about its applications and benefits. Mechanisms to monitor employee adherence to the code must be developed as well.

The *Code of Ethics* and Ethical Policy Statement of the American College of Healthcare Executives, the leading professional association of healthcare leaders, are excellent guides for practicing leaders, managers, students, consultants, and others interested in the management field (see the *Code*'s Preamble in exhibit 7.1). Many healthcare organizations also have a corporate code of ethics or statement or a corporate responsibility program.

Several excellent examples can be found online. Premier Health posts a description of its commitment to integrity and ethics on its website at www.premierhealth.com/Our-Community/Premier-Mission/Integrity-and-Ethics/. Similarly, Ascension Health's comprehensive Corporate Responsibility Program can be found at www.ascensionhealth.org/assets/docs/CorpRespBrochure.pdf.

Some organizations create ethics statements because of regulatory requirements and corporate compliance programs. However, an increasing number of healthcare organizations have put in place robust codes of ethics because doing so is the right thing and is beneficial to the enterprise as a whole.

Exhibit 7.1 Preamble to ACHE's *Code of Ethics*

The purpose of the *Code of Ethics* of the American College of Healthcare Executives is to serve as a standard of conduct for members. It contains standards of ethical behavior for healthcare executives in their professional relationships. These relationships include colleagues, patients or others served; members of the healthcare executive's organization and other organizations; the community; and society as a whole.

The *Code of Ethics* also incorporates standards of ethical behavior governing individual behavior, particularly when that conduct directly relates to the role and identity of the healthcare executive.

The fundamental objectives of the healthcare management profession are to maintain or enhance the overall quality of life, dignity and well-being of every individual needing healthcare service and to create a more equitable, accessible, effective and efficient healthcare system.

Healthcare executives have an obligation to act in ways that will merit the trust, confidence and respect of healthcare professionals and the general public. Therefore, healthcare executives should lead lives that embody an exemplary system of values and ethics.

In fulfilling their commitments and obligations to patients or others served, healthcare executives function as moral advocates and models. Since every management decision affects the health and well-being of both individuals and communities, healthcare executives must carefully evaluate the possible outcomes of their decisions. In organizations that deliver healthcare services, they must work to safeguard and foster the rights, interests and prerogatives of patients or others served.

The role of moral advocate requires that healthcare executives take actions necessary to promote such rights, interests and prerogatives.

Being a model means that decisions and actions will reflect personal integrity and ethical leadership that others will seek to emulate.

Source: Reprinted from American College of Healthcare Executives (2011).

Write a Personal Code of Ethics

Writing a personal code of ethics, or credo, serves two purposes: (1) to declare the values important to the person, and (2) to guide decision making and prioritizing when difficult issues come up. In adopting a credo, a leader should consider how other people perceive her behaviors and actions. As one CEO simply puts it, "What do others think of you?"

Here are questions to ponder when developing a personal code of ethics:

- What does integrity mean to me?
- What do I value?
- What do I stand for?
- What am I willing to compromise or not compromise?

Committing to abide by this code of ethics is the next step. This commitment entails weighing the cost of not being ethical. The cost is significant, as illustrated by leaders in the field who have been caught peddling dubious schemes, misappropriating funds, or generally behaving badly. Here are questions to consider in this regard:

- What damage will this situation cause to my loved ones? To my career and livelihood? To my reputation in the community?
- Is the payoff worth everything I have worked hard to build?

Tell the Truth, and Do Not Exaggerate

In the strict ethical sense, telling the truth and not exaggerating are the same. Many people, however, differentiate between the two. The argument for the difference is that telling the truth means telling no lies. On the other hand, exaggerating means stretching the truth to achieve a certain outcome or reaction.

For many, including healthcare executives, the latter has become accepted, commonplace practice. Many executives overestimate, engage in hyperbole, embellish the facts, provide misquotes, twist the truth, and overstate (or understate) their contribution or responsibility to fit their needs. Whether discussing budget or organizational performance, many communications are filled with subjective stretches of reality. Consider the following simple, but powerful, comments that are often rhetorical overstatements:

> Claiming more credit than you're due is yet another way we may fool ourselves about the moral virtue of our own decision making.
>
> —Richard L. Hughes, Robert C. Ginnett, and Gordon J. Curphy (2015)

- "We have cut all the fat out of our budgets. All that remains is absolutely necessary."
- "I have told the team that many, many times. They must not be hearing me."
- "I don't think I can cut any deeper—it will hurt patient care."
- "Everyone is very upset about this."

How many times have you heard these or similar statements, and how many times have you fully believed them?

Do As You Say

Become known as a leader who follows through. Often, integrity is measured less by failures in significant areas and more by the lack of follow-up on minor items. If a promise is made, it should be honored. One leader describes it as having a high "say–do" ratio.

Use Power Appropriately

Effective leaders are acutely aware that power can be used for good or bad. They understand the sources of their power, and they use it judiciously. Unfortunately, ineffective leaders and some new executives wield their power to attempt to gain respect, prestige, and favors.

Admit Mistakes

Admitting mistakes is a noble, impressive act. However, too many leaders believe that such an admission weakens their authority. The opposite is true. Power is not incrementally earned by being perfect all the time. Instead, power is bestowed on leaders by their followers. Followers can agree that an admission of fault serves to increase their leader's power.

March to the Beat of Your Own Drum

A clear understanding of and commitment to personal values is a leader's greatest defense against the temptation of following a negative example. An executive who is guided first and foremost by her own ethical standards, not by popular opinion or practice, behaves and performs with integrity. This type of leader does not need to beat her drum loudly to gain followers; people will follow naturally.

> Leaders face dilemmas that require choices between competing sets of values and priorities, and the best leaders recognize and face them with a commitment to doing what is right, not just what is expedient.
>
> — Richard L. Hughes, Robert C. Ginnett, and Gordon J. Curphy (2015)

Be Trustworthy

In their book *Judgment*, Tichy and Bennis (2007, 84) state, "Leading with character gives the wise leader clear-cut advantages. They are easier to trust and follow; they honor commitments and promises; their word and behavior match; they are always engaged in and by the world; they are open to reflective 'backtalk'; they can admit errors and learn from their mistakes."

Author Stephen M. R. Covey (2013) describes trust as the key way to avoid being viewed with suspicion; as such, trust reflects the essence of eth- ics and integrity. A leader is only as effective as the support that his followers grant him. Gaining that support is not possible if the leader does not earn others' trust and loyalty.

> Neither shall you allege the example of the many as an excuse for doing wrong.
>
> —Exodus 23:2

Manage Expense Accounts Judiciously

Leaders must require approvals for all reimbursements, especially for petty cash funds. This simple system of fund management does not create more bureaucracy, prevents temptation, and ensures that no one can question whether fund violation occurred.

Seasoned leaders agree that mismanagement of expenses is a common occurrence because it is so easy to overlook.

CONCLUSION

One of the greatest compliments to a leader is when others recognize her integrity and ethical uprightness. Ethics and integrity are always necessary ingredients in leadership. Leaders become great leaders when they follow their own moral instincts. Doing so focuses them in times of uncertainty, strengthening their resolve to do right no matter what.

Self-Evaluation Questions

❑ What would others say about my integrity? About my ethics?

❑ Does integrity really mean that much to me? How many times have I not followed through? Not done

(continued)

(continued from previous page)

what I said I would do? Not gotten back to someone when I promised I would?

❑ As the old saying goes, "Actions speak louder than words." How do I stack up against this saying?

❑ Do I appropriately use the power granted to me?

❑ Have I ever cut corners and behaved in an ethically questionable manner?

Cases

Case 7.1

Jennifer Park, the chief financial officer of a hospital, is preparing for the year-end financial audit. She knows that several items in the books will draw the attention of the auditors. She meets with the CEO, Rob Cortez, to explain the situation. Rob responds, "Make certain that there are no comments in the audit. The audit has to be clean because the chair is new, and he won't tolerate an audit adjustment. Do whatever it takes."

Case 7.1 Questions

1. What is the implication of Rob's instruction to Jennifer?

2. What could happen behind the scenes if Jennifer follows Rob's order? If she does not follow his order?

Case 7.2

After checking references, Jerrod D'Amato, the human resources manager at a hospital, finds out that Cheryl Johnson, the number one candidate for a critical care nursing position, was fired for absenteeism at her last job. Because the position has to be filled immediately and this discovery will only slow down the process, Jerrod chooses to withhold the information from the hiring nurse manager. He does discuss the issue with Cheryl, who tells him she was going through a tough time but is now ready for a new start. Jerrod thinks that Cheryl deserves a fair chance and that her qualifications far outweigh the problems she had.

Case 7.2 Questions
1. Is Jerrod right or wrong? Explain your reasoning.
2. Is there a difference between "need to know" information and "nice to know" information?

REFERENCES

American College of Healthcare Executives. 2011. *ACHE Code of Ethics*. Amended November 14. www.ache.org/abt_ache/code.cfm.

Burns, J. M. 1978. *Leadership*. New York: Harper & Row.

Covey, S. R. 2013. *The 7 Habits of Highly Successful People: Powerful Lessons in Personal Change*, 25th anniversary ed. New York: Simon and Schuster.

Hughes, R. L., R. C. Ginnett, and G. J. Curphy. 2015. *Leadership: Enhancing the Lessons of Experience*, 8th ed. Burr Ridge, IL: McGraw-Hill Education.

Kouzes, J. M., and B. Z. Posner. 2012. *The Leadership Challenge: How to Make Extraordinary Things Happen in Organizations*, 5th ed. San Francisco: Jossey-Bass.

Northouse, P. G. 2016. *Leadership: Theory and Practice*, 7th ed. Los Angeles: SAGE Publications.

Palanski, M. E., and F. J. Yammarino. 2007. "Integrity and Leadership: Clearing the Conceptual Confusion." *European Management Journal* 25 (3): 171–84.

Tichy, N. M., and W. G. Bennis. 2007. *Judgment: How Winning Leaders Make Great Calls*. New York: Portfolio.

SUGGESTED READINGS

Bass, B., and P. Steidlmeier. 1999. "Ethics, Character, and Authentic Transformational Leadership Behavior." *Leadership Quarterly* 10 (2): 181–217.

Gardner, W. L., C. C. Cogliser, K. M. Davis, and M. P. Dickens. 2011. "Authentic Leadership: A Review of the Literature and Research Agenda." *Leadership Quarterly* 22 (6): 1120–45.

Greenbaum, R. L., M. J. Quade, and J. Bonner. 2015. "Why Do Leaders Practice Amoral Management? A Conceptual Investigation of the Impediments to Ethical Leadership." *Organizational Psychology Review* 5 (1): 26–49.

Manz, C. C., V. Anand, M. Joshi, and K. P. Manz. 2008. "Emerging Paradoxes in Executive Leadership: A Theoretical Interpretation of the Tensions Between Corruption and Virtuous Values." *Leadership Quarterly* 19 (3): 385–92.

Storr, L. 2004. "Leading with Integrity: A Qualitative Research Study." *Journal of Health Organization and Management* 18 (6): 415–34.

CHAPTER 8

Interpersonal Connection

*Bad leaders perpetrate terrible misery
on those subject to their domain.*

—Robert Hogan and Robert B. Kaiser (2005)

ARTHUR ONLY HAD a reputation for being a great IT (information technology) manager at his health system. He was on many task forces and assigned the lead on the critical electronic health record (EHR) conversion. Arthur, who has an MBA and a PhD in information technology, applied for the chief information officer (CIO) position when its incumbent retired. He got the job, beating other equally qualified but more experienced candidates. This promotion to CIO pleased many people at the organization, but it was surprising given that Arthur was a middle manager—not necessarily next in line for the job. Among employees, the situation has become a favorite topic of discussion.

EMPLOYEE A. How did Arthur do it, landing a big CIO job so fast? He never managed budgets or led a department. He never worked directly with senior management. Granted, he was heavily involved in the EHR conversion, but I can say the same for a lot of managers here, and they're not moving up the ladder.

EMPLOYEE B. My cousin runs a large IT outsourcing firm. The turnover in those companies is very high. People frequently leave for more money, and worker loyalty is nonexistent. Somehow, though, at my cousin's firm the turnover is low, although the employees could get so much more money if they worked somewhere else.

EMPLOYEE A. Those people must be crazy!

EMPLOYEE B. Maybe so, but my cousin is an ideal boss. He sets aside time during the day to visit his employees to listen to their concerns and input. He asks about their families, and he encourages them to take classes or go back to school to advance their careers. He respects their work, and he personally thanks them for their contributions. His employees feel welcomed in his office, and they know he puts people before numbers, so they are not afraid to approach him. He is humble, supportive, and helpful. Doesn't my cousin sound like Arthur? Don't you think people would prefer to work for someone like him over someone whose main focus is always money and business?

THE HEALTHCARE SYSTEM is the true industry of the people. No other field witnesses human afflictions, from diseases of the body to ailments of the spirit; hosts the most basic human need (interaction at the most inopportune moments); and serves as the most common human thread (everyone needs healthcare). Because of these truths, people—patients, employees, physicians, volunteers, contractors, communities—are the critical factor in organizational success.

The irony is that, though leading healthcare organizations find that improving relationships with their employees and patients is the key to excellence, most still focus on financial factors to measure

success. Every organization has an annual financial audit, but only a few conduct annual human
resources audits or even define what these human
resources audits might be. Almost every board of
trustees has a finance committee, but not all have
human resources committees. Most organizations
have balanced scorecards, but the financial portion of these scorecards receives the most time and
attention.

> Leadership is a reciprocal relationship between those who choose to lead and those who decide to follow. Any discussion of leadership must attend to the dynamics of this relationship.
>
> —James M. Kouzes and Barry Z. Posner (1993)

In his well-known book *Good to Great*, Jim Collins (2001, 36) writes about the Level 5 leader. This
person "builds enduring greatness through a paradoxical blend of
personal humility and professional will." This type of leader puts
people first (i.e., "gets the right people on the bus") and vision and
strategy second. Financial success then follows this principle.

This chapter reiterates the significance of having people skills—a
value so subtle that it can be easily undermined but so powerful that
it can make or break an organization.

PEOPLE SKILLS

Leaders who have people skills are marked by a profound respect
for the character of others and a deep faith in their potential, which
is why they enjoy being with people and interact well with them.
Often, the primary deciding factor in an executive search is the
candidate's "chemistry" or ability to "blend" well with others, as
illustrated in the vignette. Although almost all organizations place
good people skills at the top of their recruitment requirement lists,
they do not emphasize the importance of this attribute to their existing employees and do not provide appropriate tools for measuring
it. Exhibit 8.1 lists definitions of "good people skills," as noted by
healthcare leaders.

The backbone of people skills is reciprocity, because without it no interaction or relationship occurs. Every healthy

Exhibit 8.1 Definitions of "Good People Skills"

- "Practices active listening, and internalizes what others say so that she can reflect on it"

- "Is comfortable with his own humanity and readily admits mistakes and apologizes when necessary"

- "Is clear about her stance on an issue but respects others' perspectives"

- "Exhibits warmth, caring, and concern"

- "Has an air of genuineness and trustworthiness"

- "Gets along well with others"

- "Is open, is approachable, and cares about developing and sustaining strong relationships"

relationship—personal or professional—is marked by a mutual exchange, a quid pro quo of sorts. This exchange strengthens the bond and encourages its duration. Nonresponsive, uninvolved rank-and-file employees can discourage even the most interactive leader.

THE CONCEPT IN PRACTICE

The following are ways to enhance interpersonal connections.

Listen

Many leaders are leaders because they are the ones in the know. For example, subject matter experts are designated to lead an initiative because of their knowledge and experience, not because of their ability to guide a group. Unfortunately, most of these leaders do too much talking, especially with subordinates, but not enough listening.

Hearing is easy because it is merely mechanical. Barring physical problems, we can all hear without exerting much effort. Listening, on the other hand, is a process that demands not only patience, time, energy, and respect but also an emotional and intellectual response. That is, listening is not (or should not be) a passive activity. In healthcare, many concerns are not articulated, if verbalized at all. Leaders must then listen more carefully to discover the root of a problem, and they must never assume the incorrect cliché "no news is good news."

Although listening is one of the most difficult tasks to master, especially in a high-stress, fast-paced environment, it is a critical skill. Exhibit 8.2 presents some techniques for improving listening.

Exhibit 8.2 How to Enhance Listening Skills

Ask a lot of questions. Be aware that the tone of your voice and the content of your questions can reveal your personal bias or opinion.

Ask clarifying questions. Do not assume the answers.

Restate the answers. Prevent misunderstanding by repeating or rephrasing in front of the person what he said.

Be open-minded. People will tell you less if they feel you are judgmental.

Be receptive to bad news. Leaders who cannot take negative news are intimidating for the wrong reasons. "Don't kill the messenger" may sound trite, but it is wise advice for every executive.

Minimize interruptions. Talking over people, acting distracted, taking phone calls, answering e-mails, and checking or posting on social media or websites are antithetical to good listening. Schedule a time for the discussion, and focus while it is happening.

Seek suggestions. Doing so sends a signal of respect and often encourages others to provide you more information.

Involve others in the conversation. Ask those who are quiet for their thoughts; their perspectives often get lost in the discussion.

Show Respect

In *Lions Don't Need to Roar,* author D. A. Benton (1992, 12) suggests that "sincerity and positive regard are two things that just can't be faked, and you need both to deal with people effectively." When asked what bothers them most about senior management, many employees state that leaders do not appreciate what they do "in the trenches." Often, this sort of observation means that executives do not make an effort to visit the units in which services are delivered; hence, they do not understand the stresses and challenges that frontline staff face on a regular basis. When leaders are absent, they cannot even thank, let alone become familiar with, those who do the work.

Strong leaders have great respect for others. They solicit ideas, share pertinent information, encourage participation in organizational initiatives and activities, show regard for others' well-being, and recognize their hard work, among many other actions. As discussed in chapter 6, "Respect is the value that multiplies the desire of both the leader and follower to work harder and deliver consistently excellent performance."

Save Time for Staff

The workday of an average healthcare executive is hectic, leaving him little time for unscheduled interactions with his direct supervisees and other staff. As a result, he can be viewed as unapproachable—someone who is too important to mingle with the rank and file.

Scheduled employee events (e.g., staff meetings, picnics, organizational socials, award luncheons, retreats, holiday parties) are ideal for a busy executive to attend. They give the leader an opportunity to connect with many people, including staff, physicians, community members, and even patients and their families.

Manage Perceptions

Perception is more important than reality because people will believe what they imagine to be true, even if it is not the actual truth. Otara (2011, 21) writes, "What people often observe or assess as your ability to be a leader and your effectiveness becomes their perception, which in turn becomes reality." Lee and I feel that managing perception is so important that we dedicate an entire chapter to it in our book *The Healthcare Leader's Guide to Actions, Awareness, and Perception* (Dye and Lee 2016).

For example, the firing of a popular manager can set off a thousand impressions, most of which would be incorrect. Specifically, it could create irrational fears or breed gossip, which could harm the culture. In this scenario, ignoring the reaction is not an option. Giving the pat "it's a confidential issue" statement is not an option either.

What leaders could do, instead, is offer the most plausible explanation to minimize the perception that someone is hiding something. In this age of more transparent leadership, employees do not tolerate secrecy and lies. The more they perceive a cover-up or wrongdoing (true or not), the more they develop a distrust for their leaders.

Leaders also have to manage perceptions about their jobs. Expensive lunches, dedicated parking spots, and other privileges send the message that leaders are more valued by the organization. Although such perks do get offered in healthcare and other industries, they are not common. When leaders receive (and accept) these perks, they must avoid the perception of any conflict of interest, which is something they expect employees to do as well.

> No matter how ambitious, capable, clear-thinking, competent . . . and witty you are, if you don't relate well to other people, you won't make it. No matter how professionally competent, financially adept, and physically solid you are, without an understanding of human nature, a genuine interest in the people around you, and the ability to establish personal bonds with them, you are severely limited in what you can achieve.
>
> —D. A. Benton (1992)

Recognize Others

Some leaders try to promote their own accomplishments by suggesting that they, rather than the people who report to them, have done the good work. People-oriented leaders behave in the opposite manner—they highlight the skills and achievements of others, particularly their own staff members. They understand that leaders are measured by the successes of their teams or followers. Therefore, the more recognition the team members receive, the higher the leader is elevated and the greater the rewards to the team as a whole.

Manage and Channel Emotions Appropriately

Many leaders create problems for themselves by losing their temper and showing the negative side of their personality. Although everyone needs to vent, leaders must be careful not to lose control because uncontrolled emotions render them unprofessional, ineffective, helpless, and feared—qualities that impede genuine, equal interactions.

Moods—whether positive or negative—must be managed. Moodiness is usually seen as a symptom of poor mental health. If given a choice, I suspect most people would choose a constantly angry leader over a moody one because no guesswork is involved with the former.

Leaders who are in control of their emotions have good people skills. They remain calm in tense situations and focused in chaotic times. As a result, they are approachable to everyone. Exhibit 8.3 presents tips on managing emotions.

Smile and Be Courteous

Many leaders may deem this suggestion silly; however, stories abound in executive search circles about executives who seem unapproachable because they are curt or do not smile. Zig Ziglar, a very successful

Exhibit 8.3 How to Manage Emotions

Listen first, react second. By listening attentively to what is being said (e.g., suggestion, feedback, criticism, praise), you are delaying your natural impulse to react. True listening demands concentration, so it deflects attention and slows reaction time.

Change your mind-set and attitude. The workplace is not a battleground, regardless of the many "bullets" you must dodge in the course of the day. Therefore, do not prepare for any kind of battle, as doing so encourages negative and survivalist thinking.

Count to ten. If listening and having a positive attitude do not work, simply count to ten. This passing of time may dull the edges of your emotional response.

Cut off your anger as quickly as possible. Anger can be the biggest obstruction to reducing the charged nature of tense interpersonal situations.

Separate feelings from facts. Base discussions (or even arguments) on facts, not emotions or biases.

Be aware of your feelings' influence on your behavior. Realize that they can harm your judgment and abilities.

---

sales trainer and author, is well known for teaching and coaching executives about the power of a smile.

Visual, nonverbal cues communicate a leader's comfort with other people. For example, steady eye contact (without glaring or leering), smiling, and a relaxed posture send the message that a person is warm, caring, and friendly. These leaders create an atmosphere of trust and respect, where staff can state their opinions and not fear the repercussions.

Focus on the Needs of Followers

"Take care of them and they will take of you" is a phrase that echoes the most basic way a leader can develop and maintain strong interpersonal connections with followers. Good executives do not take their staff's loyalty for granted, so they strive to get to know these individuals. They understand the significance of being fair, providing worthwhile or meaningful work in a safe environment, and learning what matters most to people's professional and personal lives.

The enormous changes in healthcare—from the shift to pay for value to the increased complexities of managing larger and more intricate organizations—have taken a toll on workers and caused the public to be concerned about the cost, coverage, and quality of healthcare. On top of these challenges, workers have endured large-scale downsizing and displacement, service cuts, and reorganization. At times such as these, employees must feel and know that their leaders are representing their best interest, and doing so well.

Show Compassion

A basic understanding of life's challenges and empathy for people's experiences underlies compassionate leadership. Northouse (2016, 200) indicates that compassion "refers to being sensitive to the plight of others, opening one's self to others, and being willing to help them."

For example, many Catholic hospitals have maintained high employee morale and commitment. While the number of nuns serving in hospitals has greatly contracted, those who have worked in these organizations will attest to the influence of the nuns in instilling compassion and concern for people.

Eliminate Childish, Unprofessional Behavior

Yelling, slamming doors, constantly complaining, gossiping, ignoring and then insulting others, bragging, and showing off are just some of the inappropriate behaviors that dishearten even the most patient peer or subordinate. Leaders who are secure with themselves and their position, status, and influence do not commit acts that disparage, belittle, or discredit others. Such behaviors breed intolerance, fear, low morale, poor productivity, secrecy, high turnover, and a dysfunctional culture.

Be Optimistic

Optimism or hope, while difficult to define, can be a powerful motivator of good behavior. Leaders who have great interpersonal skills are eternal optimists. They inspire and encourage people to do their best. They rally projects that are languishing or behind schedule. They reinvigorate interest in smart but forgotten suggestions or decisions. They support innovation, action, and teamwork. Northouse (2016, 204) describes optimism as the "cognitive process of viewing situations from a positive light and having favorable expectations about the future." In many leadership situations, optimism is what gets staff focused and energized. Garman and I write that leaders "have more of an effect on staff motivation than they may realize; it is therefore an area that separates high-performing leaders from average performers"(Dye and Garman 2015, 114).

Dr. Stephen Mansfield, FACHE (2016), president and CEO of Methodist Health System in Dallas, opines,

> One of the most powerful emotions leaders can instill within their organization and among their organizational followers is hope. Hope, in an organizational context, is the dynamic intersection of optimism (individual and organizational will-power) and determination or persistence in the face of adversity (individual or organizational way-power). As a measurable construct, it has been demonstrated in the literature that higher-hope organizations also have workforces that exhibit higher employee satisfaction and retention likelihood, as well

as many other positive attributes, versus their lower-hope organizational counterparts.

Being optimistic or hopeful can be learned, and it can become an imperative for leaders during a difficult time, such as a financial downturn; reorganization because of a merger, an acquisition, or budget cuts; mass layoff; unionization; and staff shortage. Of course, optimism and hope are not enough to stem the tide of workplace change or to fix the problem itself. However, it can do a lot to improve attitudes and mind-set.

Practice the Golden Rule

In the wildly popular book *All I Really Need to Know I Learned in Kindergarten,* author Robert Fulghum (1988) repeated simple lessons from childhood that resonated with people from all walks of life: Share everything. Play fair. Don't hit people. Put things back where you found them. Clean up your own mess. Don't take things that aren't yours. Say you're sorry when you hurt somebody. And so on.

The genesis of this book was Fulghum's experience with writing a personal credo (see chapter 7 for a discussion on creating a personal code of ethics). In an increasingly cynical world, these "golden rules" may be deemed corny or unimaginative, but consider this: Healthcare fraud, including highly reported white-collar crime by health system chiefs, is almost always committed by those who have never understood the meaning of "don't take things that aren't yours." The same can be said of hospital leaders who opted not to apologize to victims when a medical error caused harm or death. Studies indicate that simple apologies could prevent a costly malpractice suit. On the other hand, no leader who has "played fair" (i.e., was accountable, transparent) can be accused of wrongdoing.

For the past ten years, I have used an adaptation of Fulghum's lessons, which I share in exhibit 8.4.

Exhibit 8.4 My Take on Fulghum's Kindergarten Lessons

1. Keep your organization simple—its mission, its rules, its bureaucracy, its structure. Be sure that everyone knows why the organization is in existence—and what their roles and goals are.

2. Ensure that authority is clearly understood in the organization.

3. Make sure that everyone knows her job and gets it done.

4. Take time occasionally to recognize the fact that the job did get done (celebrate, celebrate).

5. Treat everyone with respect, dignity, and fairness.

6. Have a reason for what you do.

7. Do not be afraid to say "no," but give a reason behind the "no."

8. Communicate effectively—and then communicate some more. Share information.

9. Hire right. Make hiring a top priority.

10. Be honest; be ethical.

11. Practice servant leadership.

12. Set clear expectations, give feedback more than once per year, and listen when you give feedback.

13. Listen some more.

14. Work together in teams—people really prefer it that way.

15. Be kind to your teammates.

16. Admit mistakes.

17. Understand and appreciate the fact that when you are in a leadership position, you have a lot of benefits and perks that the rank and file do not.

Foster Employee Engagement

Since the second edition of this book, the concept of employee engagement has garnered a large following. At the time of this revision, a Google search for "employee engagement" returned more than 23 million results. However, Gallup (2016) reports that 87 percent of employees are not engaged at work and argues that the scale of the problem constitutes a crisis with long-term implications for the global economy. Some observers may believe that employee engagement in healthcare is higher than in other industries because of the service-oriented nature of healthcare work. Nonetheless, even if the percentage of disengaged people was half that of general industry, there is concern for healthcare leaders.

Moreover, Hogan and Kaiser (2005, 175) report that "estimates of the base rate for managerial incompetence in corporate life range from 30% to 75%; a recent review reported the average estimate to be 50%." This finding led to their now-famous proclamation: "Bad leaders perpetrate terrible misery on those subject to their domain" (169). Could it be more evident that much of this misery is caused by poor interpersonal skills? Gruman and Saks (2011, 125) comment that "managers can encourage employee engagement by improving manager-employee communication and creating an environment where employees feel valued." Clearly, this outcome requires strong interpersonal skills.

CONCLUSION

Leadership is about building and maintaining relationships. The effectiveness of managing personal interactions is tied to how much leaders care about being and working with others. Many years ago, the chair of a health administration graduate program warned me: "If you want to thrive in this business, you really have to love working with and around people. If you don't have a passion for that, go into another field." I cannot say it better.

Self-Evaluation Questions

❏ What does "people are our greatest asset" mean to me?

❏ Have I ever put other people down?

❏ Has anyone ever described me as a people person? Was this a source of pride for me?

❏ Has anyone ever described me as a good listener?

Cases

Case 8.1

James White has just finished a meeting with Tina Garr, his vice president, when he runs into Mary Briones, a peer departmental manager, in the hallway.

MARY. You're frowning. What's wrong?

JAMES. Nothing. I'm fine.

MARY. You look stressed. You don't seem like the regular enthusiastic James I know. Do you want to come into my office to talk about it?

JAMES. Keep this between us, but Tina is impossible to read. Sometimes she's warm and approachable. Other times, she acts as if I'm a stranger. I just tried to discuss with her my desire to take on more responsibility, because I just earned a master's degree and I've worked here for four years. I wanted her advice on what I could do to get promoted.

MARY. Those are valid questions. What did she say?

(continued)

(continued from previous page)

JAMES. She said, "You have too many projects right now. You shouldn't even be thinking of moving up." No explanation, no sugar coating. Then she said she had to go to another meeting. That's when I left.

MARY. No wonder you look dejected. Is there anything I can do to help?

Case 8.1 Questions

1. How could Tina have better handled the situation?

2. Is Mary displaying the interpersonal skills of a strong leader? How will these skills help James?

Case 8.2

Rosemary Brezinski, a veteran chief nursing officer, is the new president of a rapidly growing system hospital. Most of her impressive career has been spent in large tertiary organizations known for research and medical innovations. Her new position is a significant promotion. She is now responsible for leading the hospital's response to its recent 10 percent growth in patient volume; improving morale and collaboration among managers, staff, and physicians; and planning and implementing the move of the system's teaching program to the hospital campus, something that only the senior management knows thus far.

In the first three weeks on the job, Rosemary has held several meetings with her senior management team and leadership groups in the hospital. She has distributed to these leaders a detailed, 80-item list of priorities that will serve as the team's agenda for the next 18 months. She has informed them that she will assign each priority to an individual or a group. Her message to everyone has been consistent since the beginning of her tenure at the hospital: "I have never failed in the past. I expect that we will make these changes happen on time and on budget." She has not spoken to the medical staff or the frontline employees.

Case 8.2 Questions
1. What interpersonal connection mistakes has Rosemary made so far?
2. How do you think the staff (including the physicians and managers) feel about her style?
3. Will her mandates for change work?

REFERENCES

Benton, D. A. 1992. *Lions Don't Need to Roar: Using the Leadership Power of Professional Presence to Stand Out, Fit In, and Move Ahead.* New York: Warner Books.

Collins, J. 2001. *Good to Great: Why Some Companies Make the Leap . . . and Others Don't.* New York: HarperCollins.

Covey, S. R. 1992. *Principle-Centered Leadership.* New York: Free Press.

Dye, C. F., and A. N. Garman. 2015. *Exceptional Leadership: 16 Critical Competencies for Healthcare Leaders,* 2nd ed. Chicago: Health Administration Press.

Dye, C. F., and B. D. Lee. 2016. *The Healthcare Leader's Guide to Actions, Awareness, and Perception,* 3rd ed. Chicago: Health Administration Press.

Fulghum, R. 1988. *All I Really Need to Know I Learned in Kindergarten: Uncommon Thoughts on Common Things.* New York: Villard Books.

Gallup. 2016. "The Culture of an Engaged Workplace: Q12 Engagement." Accessed March 30. www.gallup.com/services/169328/q12-employee-engagement.aspx.

Gruman, J. A., and A. M. Saks. 2011. "Performance Management and Employee Engagement." *Human Resource Management Review* 21 (2): 123–36.

Hogan, R., and R. B. Kaiser. 2005. "What We Know About Leadership." *Review of General Psychology* 9 (2): 169–80.

Kouzes, J. M., and B. Z. Posner. 1993. *Credibility: How Leaders Gain It and Lose It, Why People Demand It*. San Francisco: Jossey-Bass.

Mansfield, S. 2016. Personal communication with author, May 12.

Northouse, P. G. 2016. *Leadership: Theory and Practice*, 7th ed. Los Angeles: SAGE Publications.

Otara, A. 2011. "Perception: A Guide for Managers and Leaders." *Journal of Management and Strategy* 2 (3): 21–22.

SUGGESTED READINGS

Buch, R., G. Thompson, and B. Kuvaas. 2016. "Transactional Leader–Member Exchange Relationships and Followers' Work Performance: The Moderating Role of Leaders' Political Skill." *Journal of Leadership and Organizational Studies*. Published February 15. http://jlo.sagepub.com/content/early/2016/02/12/1548051816630227.abstract.

Collins, J. 2001. "Level 5 Leadership: The Triumph of Humility and Fierce Resolve." *Harvard Business Review* 79 (1): 66–79.

Jian, G., and F. Dalisay. 2015. "Conversation at Work: The Effects of Leader-Member Conversational Quality." *Communication Research*. Published January 8. http://crx.sagepub.com/content/early/2015/01/07/0093650214565924.abstract.

Laschinger, H. K., L. Borgogni, C. Consiglio, and E. Read. 2014. "The Effects of Authentic Leadership, Six Areas of Worklife, and Occupational Coping Self-efficacy on New Graduate Nurses' Burnout and Mental Health: A Cross-Sectional Study." *International Journal of Nursing Studies* 52 (6): 1080–89.

Tan, C.-M. 2013. *Search Inside Yourself: The Secret to Unbreakable Concentration, Complete Relaxation, and Effortless Self-Control*. New York: HarperCollins.

Uhl-Bien, M. 2006. "Relational Leadership Theory: Exploring the Social Processes of Leadership and Organizing." *Leadership Quarterly* 17 (6): 654–76.

Yeager, K. L., and J. L. Callahan. 2016. "Learning to Lead: Foundations of Emerging Leader Identity Development." *Advances in Developing Human Resources*. Published April 27. http://jlo.sagepub.com/content/early/2016/02/12/1548051816630227.abstract.

CHAPTER 9

Servant Leadership

The servant leader is servant first. . . . *It begins with the natural feeling that one wants to serve, to serve first. Then conscious choice brings one to aspire to lead. That person is sharply different from one who is* leader first, *perhaps because of the need to assuage an unusual power drive or to acquire material possessions. . . . The leader first and the servant first are two extreme types. Between them there are shadings and blends that are part of the infinite variety of human nature.*

—Robert K. Greenleaf (1970)

"WHAT IS YOUR primary role as a leader?" Sister Mary O'Hara, the president and CEO of a soon-to-open community hospital, asked her newly formed management team. The answers varied:

- Work toward our mission and vision.
- Get everyone to work cooperatively.
- Manage efficiently and effectively.
- Meet our goals and make sure our employees do their jobs.

Sister Mary responded, "All of these are good ideas. What I want you to keep in mind most of all is this: Each of you is a servant leader. By that I mean that your job is to serve those who report to you. Help them do their work, and let them help you do yours. Be humble. You do not know all the answers and you're not the experts, so seek input from others. Give credit and praise liberally, and be generous with your time regardless of how busy you become. Listen before you speak. Ask how you can lend a hand. Teach and encourage learning. I realize that some of you may have a different view of leadership than what I just laid out. But the mission of our community hospital is to serve, and that is exactly what we are going to do—we will serve each other, regardless of our titles."

The management team applauded loudly in agreement.

THE HEALTHCARE FIELD was established with a simple, altruistic purpose: to serve the public. Therefore, its leaders must subscribe to the same mission by becoming "servants" to the needs of their organizations and constituents. Servant leadership is not merely a trendy practice arising from political correctness or a cliché intonation of "following to lead"; instead, it is a management style that delivers desired outcomes, boosts morale, strengthens the organizational structure, and generates support for the leader.

According to Northouse (2016, 239), "Servant leaders make it a point to listen to their followers and develop strong long-term relationships with others. This allows leaders to understand the abilities, needs, and goals of followers, which, in turn, allows these followers to achieve their full potential." Since it was first theorized in the 1970s, servant leadership has gained a large following, including experts in management and organizational behavior such as Peter Senge, Stephen Covey, Margaret Wheatley, and Ken Blanchard. Exhibit 9.1 contrasts traditional leadership with servant leadership.

Be mindful of this, though: Servant leadership does not connote waiting for others to move to action. In fact, servant leaders are very focused on goals and improvement. Sousa and van Dierendonck

Exhibit 9.1 Traditional Leadership Versus Servant Leadership

Motivation	To Lead	To Serve
Approach	Top-down, command and control	Bottom-up, collaborative
Basis	Power and authority	Stewardship
Primary focus	Finance	People
Self-awareness	Not important	Critical
Followers	May or may not grow	Definitely will grow

(2015, 1) state, "Whereas it may be possible to speak about servant leadership as one specific way of leadership, at a deeper level . . . there seem to be two overarching encompassing dimensions: a humble service-oriented side and an action-driven side, both coexisting and complementing each other."

Also, servant leaders are role models and teachers. They set an example for others, as one CEO does: "I gave each executive in the organization a small rock and a small ceramic monkey to place on their desks. The purpose of the rock and the monkey is to help them to be always mindful of what they need to do—keep the rocks and barriers out of the way so their staff can do their jobs. And if the staff can do their jobs, they [the executives] won't put inappropriate monkeys on their back." Another CEO echoes this principle: "My job is to take away any obstacles that keep [the people who report to me] from succeeding. . . . If there's an obstacle between you and any of our targets, I need to know about it."

In essence, the success of leaders who serve depends on how well they meet their

A servant leader demonstrates the following behaviors:

1. Focuses on the needs of followers

2. Eschews selfish behavior, personal biases, and pursuit of personal ambition

3. Sincerely respects all people

4. Realizes that the contributions of followers are what enable the organization to fulfill its mission

5. Helps, encourages, and counsels followers to hone their skills and become better at their positions because doing so brings the organization closer to its goals

followers' needs. Followers are more efficient, productive, and satisfied when given autonomy, support, resources, and positive examples. As a result, they perform better than expected and grow personally and professionally. More important, they are more likely to become servant leaders themselves.

Servant leadership may be likened to transformational leadership in that both philosophies "show concern for their followers, [but] the overriding focus of the servant leader is upon service to their followers. The transformational leader has a greater concern for getting followers to engage in and support organizational objectives" (Stone, Russell, and Patterson 2003, 4).

THE CONCEPT IN PRACTICE

The following guidelines can hone a leader's servant skills.

Share Information

Sharing information freely with peers and subordinates opens communication pathways through which ideas travel. A two-way exchange of ideas signifies the leader's respect for other perspectives and trust in others' ability to contribute. Although information is power, a servant leader is disinclined to abuse the knowledge he acquires to manipulate the situation for his own good.

> A new moral principle is emerging which holds that the only authority deserving one's allegiance is that which is freely and knowingly granted by the led to the leader in response to, and in proportion to, the clearly evident servant stature of the leader.
>
> —Robert K. Greenleaf (1983)

Delegate Authority

Delegation not only increases productivity but also promotes teamwork, especially during times of crisis (although many leaders tend to take the reins when serious problems arise). In a crisis situation, servant leaders are not apprehensive about delegating authority to members of their leadership team because they have regularly included and coached them in brainstorming, problem solving, decision making, and implementation. Thus, these leaders are confident of their staff's ability to perform under great stress.

Delegating authority should be a frequent practice in healthcare organizations because the challenges and responsibilities are often too intricate for one person to handle alone. In addition, frontline staff directly face the everyday dilemmas of the workplace and therefore often have more practical and sustainable solutions than what supervisors, directors, and vice presidents can offer. Servant leaders are aware of this dynamic.

> Understanding the tools needed for effective leadership is important, and the servant leadership philosophy offers leaders the opportunity to not only understand the needs of the organization but also . . . to incorporate one of the most valuable tools necessary in making the organization effective: followers.
>
> —Amy R. Savage-Austin and Andrew Honeycutt (2011)

Live the Mission and Pursue the Vision

Most mission statements of healthcare organizations include the word *serve*. Servant leaders take their missions to heart. They ensure that the organizational vision, values, culture, strategies, and activities are consistent with the mission. They enlist others, including physicians, in establishing policies and practices that support and advance the mission.

Servant leaders are also visionaries. Being future oriented and innovative, they seek to understand past events and current realities—any factors that have an impact on the future operation of the organization. They encourage staff to participate in this visioning work, aware that such an engagement facilitates the achievement of the vision.

Support and Promote Continuing Education

All employees can pursue continuing education to enhance their professional or vocational skills, which consequently improves their job marketability. Servant leaders not only apportion organizational funds to finance staff's educational pursuits (e.g., degree programs, professional seminars, certification courses) but also provide coaching.

"Teaching moments"—occasions that give leaders the opportunity to explain an organizational decision, policy, process, practice, or stance—are an excellent way to inform and engage the staff. For example, an adverse medical event is a teaching moment wherein leaders can review safety standards, reiterate quality policies, delineate the role of staff, and exchange questions and ideas about improvement.

Most important, professional and personal development must go beyond lip service. Policies (and budget) that support continuing education must be in place. Specifically, performance expectations should include a requirement to complete a certain number of continuing education hours by the next performance review. The onus of checking up on this requirement must fall on the leader.

Provide Opportunities for Accomplishments

Servant leaders do not set up their followers to fail. Structured objectives and clear instructions help staff reach their goals and complete their assignments. Moreover, these leaders provide coaching and support when needed, but they allow employees freedom to work toward their own objectives. In doing so, staff gain mastery of their jobs, greater enjoyment from their work, confidence, new skills, and feelings of achievement. They are proud to say, "We did this ourselves." Liden and colleagues (2008) found an empirical correlation between servant leadership behaviors and employee organizational commitment.

Establish a Succession Plan

The sudden departure of a leader (voluntarily or involuntarily) can cause much chaos and uncertainty in the organization. The situation can become even worse when no succession plan is in place that details that leader's replacement. Baby boomers continue to retire, and yet many healthcare organizations have no succession plans.

Although healthcare executives are cognizant of the importance of succession planning, they do not engage in the practice readily. According to one study (Garman and Tyler 2007) that yielded 722 responses, the most frequently cited reason for not conducting succession planning was that it was not a high enough priority (46 percent). Other reasons cited were because the current CEO was too new (31 percent) and that there was no internal candidate to prepare (25 percent). In contrast, succession planning is a priority for servant leaders because their first priority is the needs of their employees, who deserve strong and dependable leadership.

Learn About the Work

When employees complain that their leaders are "out of touch," they are mostly right. Leaders cannot empathize with frontline staff if they do not understand what this work entails. Visiting the units and talking with staff are some strategies for learning the work. But leaders could go a step further by shadowing employees and interacting with patients and their families.

Servant leaders partake in these experiences, enabling them to encounter firsthand the difficulties they only hear about, to speak the language of caregivers and support staff, and to discover areas

> Being a servant may not be what many leaders had in mind when they chose to take responsibility for the vision and direction of their organization or team, but serving others is the most glorious and rewarding of all leadership tasks.
>
> —James M. Kouzes and Barry Z. Posner (1993)

for improvement. In the process, both leaders and employees get to know each other better, paving the way for mutual understanding of their distinct roles.

Mentor Others

Clearly, healthcare executives are pressed for time, and mentoring often becomes a casualty of the rush. Mentoring is a critical competency that sets apart good leaders from great ones (see Dye and Garman 2015). Servant leaders are advocates for personal and professional development. As such, they provide coaching and support continuing education.

Hold Simple Celebrations

Servant leaders are acutely aware of the morale-boosting capability of simple celebrations and praise. A round of applause during a staff meeting, an acknowledgment in an organization-wide publication or on the intranet, or a plate of cookies are small gestures that carry great weight. For example, one chief financial officer holds a pizza party for the credit and collection workers when they meet their monthly numbers. The employees are gratified and motivated to repeat their achievement.

Change the Focus of Performance Reviews

Annual or midyear performance reviews are often met with dread. The main reason for this mind-set is these assessments are essentially criticism—what mistakes were committed, what goals were not accomplished, what skills were not improved, and so on. As a result, the feedback is taken as a personal offense, not as a constructive comment. No one wants to feel attacked, so no one enjoys this type of review.

Leaders who serve are aware of this reaction, so they structure the performance evaluation differently:

- The focus is future performance, not past missteps or lost opportunities.
- Achievement of objectives is celebrated. Goals are developed with input from the employee and with consideration of the person's ability, environmental obstacles, available resources, and realistic timelines. These goals are monitored during the year.
- No blame is placed, and the factors that contributed to poor performance are discussed so that they are corrected or eliminated.
- Ongoing development is encouraged, regardless of how high the rank of the employee.

If organizational constraints do not allow for this type of progressive discussion, highly effective leaders then set aside other times to have conversations about performance and progress.

Make a Connection with Staff

Servant leaders are not aloof or detached. They maintain relationships and stay abreast of issues that affect all of their associates—staff, physicians, board members, community leaders, and peers.

Making a connection could be as simple as visiting departments or attending organizational events or as involved as getting to know the staff. Perhaps one of the best ways a leader can make a connection is by showing employees that she is one of them, as

> Whereas takers tend to be self-focused, evaluating what other people can offer them, givers are other-focused, paying more attention to what other people need from them.
>
> —Adam Grant (2013)

this example from Andrea Price, FACHE (2016)—former chair of the National Association of Health Services Executives and former member of the Board of Governors of the American College of Healthcare Executives—illustrates:

> I lead by putting people first, whether or not they report to me. It's my duty to help other people succeed, so I provide as much support, coaching, encouragement, feedback, and guidance as necessary. I also give them a chance to demonstrate their skills and knowledge so that they can become aware of their own strengths and weaknesses. I serve as a resource to my staff, readily available to address their needs. . . . There is nothing that goes on in the hospital that I am unwilling to do, regardless of my title. I have mopped spills off the floor in my suit and heels, much to the amazement of the staff. While I was rounding late one night, I met a patient who was hungry for a salad. I went to the cafeteria and prepared a salad according to how the patient wanted it. As a healthcare executive, I can't give medication, but I can get water for a patient.

CONCLUSION

Picture an organization in which everybody performs every activity with the primary intention of serving someone else. This vision seems like utopia, but it is achievable, and it starts with leaders. If subordinates feel that their leaders serve them, they will likely model that behavior toward others. As a result, service to patients will be enhanced, improving the organization's competitive advantage. As Garman and I write, "A fundamental polarity in leadership involves the balance between self-interest (what you do to serve your own needs) and selfless interest (what you do to serve the needs of others or the needs of the organization)" (Dye and Garman 2015, 17).

Self-Evaluation Questions

❑ Why am I in a leadership position?

❑ What is my leadership style? Does it place a heavy emphasis on controlling others?

❑ Does the idea of serving others make me think that I am a weak leader?

Case and Exercises

Case 9.1

Two students in an executive seminar, Rachel Goh and Jared Kaufman, explore the basis of servant leadership in class.

RACHEL. I don't buy it. The idea that servant leaders are more committed to their followers and organization sounds too religious for me. The fact is, people are, at the core, selfish. We act with self-interest, first and always.

JARED. Servant leaders are manipulative, but in a good way. Take me, for example. My staff can't get along well without me because I provide them with everything they need—from advice to tangible resources. This is a win–win situation. I support their work, and in exchange I get the results I want.

Case 9.1 Questions

Do you agree with this summation that servant leadership is (a) not possible given the selfish nature of people and (b) secretly or outwardly manipulative but harmless? Explain your answer.

Using Greenleaf's definition of this theory (see www. greenleaf.org), discuss how servant leadership can guide executives in today's healthcare environment.

(continued)

(continued from previous page)

Exercise 9.1

Servant leadership is likely to work best in an organizational culture that supports it. That is, some cultures have a high level of trust and team orientation, while others are hierarchical or rely on command-and-control principles. What types of culture can support the practice of servant leadership?

See the following websites for a discussion on organizational culture:

- http://managementhelp.org/org_thry/culture/culture.htm
- http://study.com/academy/lesson/what-is-organizational-culture-definition-characteristics.html
- www.tnellen.com/ted/tc/schein.html
- www.thercfgroup.com/files/resources/Defining-Culture-and-Organizationa-Culture_5.pdf

Exercise 9.2

Two excellent academic reviews of servant leadership are provided by Savage-Austin and Honeycutt and Sokoll. Review both and summarize their key conclusions.

Savage-Austin, A. R., and A. Honeycutt. 2011. "Servant Leadership: A Phenomenological Study of Practices, Experiences, Organizational Effectiveness, and Barriers." *Journal of Business and Economics Research* 9 (1): 49–54. www.clute institute.com/ojs/index.php/JBER/article/viewFile/939/923.

Sokoll, S. 2014. "Servant Leadership and Employee Commitment to a Supervisor." *International Journal of Leadership Studies* 8 (2): 88–104. www.regent.edu/acad/global/publications/ijls/new/vol8iss2/5-Sokoll.pdf.

REFERENCES

Dye, C. F., and A. N. Garman. 2015. *Exceptional Leadership: 16 Critical Competencies for Healthcare Executives*, 2nd ed. Chicago: Health Administration Press.

Garman, A., and J. L. Tyler. 2007. *Succession Planning Practices and Outcomes in US Hospital Systems: Final Report*. Chicago: American College of Healthcare Executives.

Grant, A. 2013. *Give and Take: A Revolutionary Approach to Success*. New York: Viking.

Greenleaf, R. K. 1983. *Servant Leadership: A Journey into the Nature of Legitimate Power and Greatness*. Mahwah, NJ: Paulist Press.

————. 1970. *The Servant as Leader*. Westfield, IN: Greenleaf Center for Servant Leadership.

Kouzes, J. M., and B. Z. Posner. 1993. *Credibility: How Leaders Gain and Lose It, Why People Demand It*. San Francisco: Jossey-Bass.

Liden, R. C., S. J. Wayne, H. Zhao, and D. Henderson. 2008. "Servant Leadership: Development of a Multidimensional Measure and Multi-level Assessment." *Leadership Quarterly* 19 (2): 161–77.

Northouse, P. G. 2016. *Leadership: Theory and Practice*, 7th ed. Los Angeles: SAGE Publications.

Price, A. 2016. Personal communication with author, May 16.

Savage-Austin, A. R., and A. Honeycutt. 2011. "Servant Leadership: A Phenomenological Study of Practices, Experiences, Organizational Effectiveness, and Barriers." *Journal of Business and Economics Research* 9 (1): 49–54.

Sousa, M., and D. van Dierendonck. 2015. "Servant Leadership and the Effect of the Interaction Between Humility, Action, and Hierarchical Power on Follower Engagement." *Journal of Business Ethics.* Published June 13. http://link.springer.com/article/10.1007/s10551-015-2725-y.

Stone, A. G., R. F. Russell, and K. Patterson. 2003. "Transformational Versus Servant Leadership: A Difference in Leader Focus." Servant Leadership Research Roundtable, School of Leadership Studies, Regents University, Virginia Beach, VA, August.

SUGGESTED READINGS

Bobbio, A., and A. M. Manganelli. 2015. "Antecedents of Hospital Nurses' Intention to Leave the Organization: A Cross Sectional Survey." *International Journal of Nursing Studies* 52 (7): 1180–92.

Newman, A., G. Schwarz, B. Cooper, and S. Sendjaya. 2015. "How Servant Leadership Influences Organizational Citizenship Behavior: The Roles of LMX, Empowerment, and Proactive Personality." *Journal of Business Ethics.* Published September. DOI 10.1007/s10551-015-2827-6.

Panaccio, A., D. J. Henderson, R. C. Liden, S. J. Waynes, and X. Cao. 2015. "Toward an Understanding of When and Why Servant Leadership Accounts for Employee Extra-Role Behaviors." *Journal of Business and Psychology* 30 (4): 657–75.

Parris, D. L., and J. W. Peachey. 2013. "A Systematic Literature Review of Servant Leadership Theory in Organizational Contexts." *Journal of Business Ethics* 113 (3): 377–93.

Swenson, S., G. Gorringe, J. Caviness, and D. Peters. 2016. "Leadership by Design: Intentional Organization Development of Physician Leaders." *Journal of Management Development* 35 (4): 549–70.

van Dierendonck, D., and I. Nuijten. 2011. "The Servant Leadership Survey: Development and Validation of a Multidimensional Measure." *Journal of Business and Psychology* 26 (3): 249–67.

VanMeter, R., L. B. Chonko, D. B. Grisaffe, and E. A. Goad. 2016. "In Search of Clarity on Servant Leadership: Domain Specification and Reconceptualization." *AMS Review* 6 (1): 59–78.

CHAPTER 10

Desire to Make a Change

Altruism is the quality that makes professionals think and act in the interest of serving the community. Without it, healthcare could become a profession of people pursuing their own interests or selfish goals, instead of a public service that everyone can rely on.

—Elizabeth J. Forrestal and Leigh W. Cellucci (2016)

S EVERAL YEARS AGO, Elaine Rostovich asked her boss Barb Valdez why she gave up overtime pay and shift differentials to become a nurse manager.

Barb answered, "The loss in pay doesn't matter to me as much as gaining the ability to make improvements around here. As a staff nurse, I couldn't change anything that was no longer working. Sure, I do a lot more paperwork and face more stress now, but it's satisfying to see that our clinical outcomes are better and our staff and patients are happier because we're now more efficient."

Barb's reasoning finally makes sense to Elaine as she listens to her mentor emphasize the importance of leading change: "Like a lot of healthcare CEOs, I entered the field because I wanted to make a difference in people's lives. This topic hasn't been researched a lot, but that desire is the true beginning of improvement. Those who have this passion work hard to make positive changes happen, and they don't do it for money, praise, or prestige. They do it because they understand that nothing is beyond improvement. They use all their resources, skills, and knowledge to accomplish their goals. They are some of the most well-informed people around, these change leaders."

THE DESIRE TO make a change is one of the most distinctive values of a strong leader. *Change makers*, as these leaders are known, are high achievers. They actively seek out flaws in the system and implement improvements. While campers abide by the rule "leave a campsite in better condition than you found it," change makers initiate upgrades even before they get to the campsite. They are proactive and innovative, and they welcome challenges.

CHARACTERISTICS OF A CHANGE MAKER

In the 1960s, motivational theorist David McClelland posited that individuals who have achievement motivation, as is the case with change makers, are likely to be goal oriented and uphold high standards of performance. These individuals are most likely to move into leadership positions because they can operate well and even flourish despite the high levels of stress and unceasing demands for long hours, critical thinking, and quick turnarounds. Such leaders also have broad strategic views. Bolman and Deal (2013, 24) state that "managers are supposed to see the big picture and look out for their organization's overall health and productivity." Moreover, Rylatt (2013) writes, "To be exceptional in influencing large-scale change requires an excellent grasp of the complexities and tensions of organizational culture and the sources of power and authority. High-performing change agents stand apart from

Our current success is the best reason to change things.

—Iwao Isomura (1998)

others by virtue of their ability to negotiate more expansive and powerful job profiles that increase their capacity to generate meaningful outcomes."

Change makers have *restless discontent*—the inability to live with the status quo. They cannot tolerate ineffective processes that force people to muddle through ill-conceived standards and processes. One CEO defines this discontent as an "ability to sense opportunities." This description is fitting, as change makers are constantly on the lookout for new ideas. The discontent peels away as areas for improvement garner attention and the need for change earns buy-in from others, especially senior management. According to Hughes, Ginnett, and Curphy (2015, 560), "Leading change is perhaps the most difficult challenge facing any leader, yet this skill may be the best differentiator of managers from leaders and of mediocre from exceptional leaders."

For many healthcare leaders, the desire to make a change has become a professional calling. This approach is evident in the rise of the quality improvement movement in healthcare, which calls for

- establishing measurable goals and standards,
- developing systems for monitoring progress toward and achieving desired outcomes,
- disseminating lessons learned,
- celebrating successes, and
- continuing improvement efforts.

THE CONCEPT IN PRACTICE
Pay Equal Attention to All Measures of Performance

In flight school, student pilots are taught how to maneuver their planes guided only by their instrument panels. This technique teaches pilots to fly safely despite hindrances that may surround them—thick fog, utter darkness, raging storms, and other conditions that impair

> **Change Makers Have Achievement Motivation**
>
> In his classic text, David McClelland (1961) posits the following attributes of high achievers:
>
> 1. They address problems rather than leave them to chance.
>
> 2. Their goals can be accomplished—neither too difficult nor too easy.
>
> 3. They are more interested in accomplishment than in rewards.
>
> 4. They seek workplaces and positions that offer ample feedback.
>
> 5. They constantly think about improvement, excellence, and perfection. They seek out organizations that will allow them to make changes.

visibility. However, some pilots tend to pay the most attention to the altimeter, which tells the position and location of the plane on the horizon. Although the altimeter is an important gauge, this instrument is not the only one a pilot should check. Trouble almost always ensues when the other critical measures are overlooked. This danger is also seen in healthcare management.

All healthcare leaders—new or seasoned—have, at one point or another, focused only on the financial report when determining the status of their organization. This tendency is understandable; after all, without funds the operation will cease to exist, an especially salient issue in an environment filled with bankruptcies and acquisitions. However, healthcare is hardly a one-dimensional enterprise. If too much priority is given to revenue, capital, debt, investment, and other elements of finance, then not enough attention is given to human resources, patient safety, clinical outcomes, quality improvement, physician relations, and the like.

Change makers understand that the organization is a system and thus needs a system-based approach. Simply put, a flaw in one component can cause damage to another, ushering in a cascading effect.

Turn Satisfied Employees into Engaged Employees

High-performing organizations tend to have highly satisfied workers. However, satisfaction does not lead to engagement. Many happy employees walk in and out of their jobs daily without a desire to participate in the activities that cause their happiness. They may ignore areas that could use improvement because they think bringing about change is not part of their job responsibilities.

Employee engagement has been defined many ways, but practically all definitions indicate emotional connection or attachment to the work and goals of an organization. Engagement is neither satisfaction nor happiness. The fact is that employees can be satisfied and happy and yet not engaged. Harter and Adkins (2015) put it simply, stating that engaged employees are "involved in, enthusiastic about, and committed to their work and workplace." Gallup (2016) finds that "when employees are engaged, they are passionate, creative, and entrepreneurial, and their enthusiasm fuels growth. These employees are emotionally connected to the mission and purpose of their work." Exhibit 10.1 describes the linkage between employees' level of engagement and desire to make changes.

Note that more and more human resources firms are conducting employee engagement (as opposed to employee satisfaction) surveys. This practice signals a shift in mind-set: Good employees have much to contribute to the viability of the organization. Seeking participation from employees could also bring out the latent change makers among them. Jim Haudan, the CEO of Root, emphasizes that for change

---

Exhibit 10.1 Linkage Between Employee Engagement and Desire to Make Changes

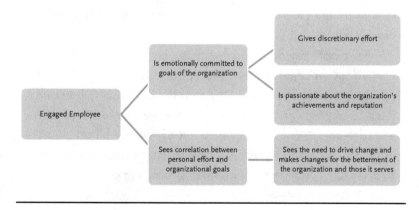

---

and improvement to be fully executed, employees at all levels must be given the opportunity to internalize the thinking and rationale behind the strategy. Haudan (2016) reiterates that the most effective leaders create environments where employees are highly engaged.

> Real engagement is multidimensional and can be effortless, natural, and magnetic. Throughout the past 25 years of working with businesses, [I have found] four proven approaches that truly drive powerful employee engagement have emerged. These approaches frame employees as customers and see engagement through the eyes of the people we serve as leaders. They help people feel enthralled, drawn in, and connected in a compelling and sustained way to the work that they do. They quickly become the foundation, or roots, for engaging your people. [These approaches] include (1) helping them feel like they're part of something bigger than themselves, (2) giving people a sense of belonging, (3) feeling like they're on a meaningful journey, and (4) showing people their contributions are making a difference.
>
> Part of that engagement process comes in helping people understand the big picture of what the company is trying to achieve—arriving at the same conclusion on their own—and then recognizing their own role in helping drive those results. Most leaders leverage data and a show-and-tell process to engage people in the company strategy. But look at the following image [see exhibit 1.2 in chapter 1], which combines visuals, data, and stories.
>
> While both the data and the image convey similar information about an organization, which one are you most likely to remember after one hour? One month? One year? Now think back to any PowerPoint or memo that you've received from a leader about the strategy or a list of ten key bullet points. How much of an impression do the words make compared to a visual? Imagine that, instead of sending out a memo to introduce your people to a new initiative, your organization rolled out a new strategy by holding small group discussions

built around an image like this one. This is the power of metaphor, visualization, and discussion to truly drive engagement.

Be Objective Driven and Progress Oriented

Change makers are passionate about setting objectives for both professional and organizational purposes. Doing so helps them measure the effectiveness of their performance, decisions, and activities. Many leaders fail to set clear goals, delaying or impeding progress and achievement and frustrating those involved.

In addition, change makers admit that even the best organizations (and employees) must evolve with the times. Thus, they push to move forward, tracking their steps along the way with available measurement tools. SMART—specific, measurable, attainable, realistic, and timely—is still the best strategy for setting goals, although it is now more than two decades old (see Kouzes and Posner 1993 for more information). SMART goals allow organizations to focus simultaneously on the present and the future.

> Developing vision means that you see the future clearly, anticipate large-scale and local changes that will affect the organization and its environment, are able to project the organization into the future and envision multiple potential scenarios or outcomes, have a broad way of looking at trends, and are able to design competitive strategies and plans based on future possibilities.
>
> —Carson F. Dye and Andrew N. Garman (2015)

Welcome Change

Change makers enjoy new challenges and are not afraid of taking risks. For them, change is a normal part of leadership and presents opportunities. As such, they prefer to err on the side of overstudying or overanalyzing trends than to be misinformed. Being prepared serves as a defense against the unknown or sudden change that seems unmanageable.

The fear of making the wrong decision is endemic in healthcare. On the clinical side, an error could result in injury or death and subsequently costly and drawn-out lawsuits. On the business side, an error could result in loss of customers and consequently revenue. Certainly, cautious decisions are in order.

However, this general rule does not mean risks should not be taken. Progress and innovation—two words that most leaders would like to be associated with—are not driven by fear. They are possible only with leaps of faith, albeit calculated.

Celebrate Accomplishments

As discussed in chapter 9, people enjoy celebrations, especially if they highlight the product of their hard work. A celebration of accomplishments not only embodies the joy, relief, and pride of the team, it also underscores the gratitude of the leaders. People who are able to see that their efforts have made a difference and are appreciated are likely to repeat their performance in the future and feel empowered. Empowerment is a strong motivation because it makes people feel in control and valued.

Celebrations may also be used to improve morale. For example, one executive organizes a monthly "Breakfast of Champions" for employees. Individuals and departments who make progress toward goals are recognized during the program and given a box of Wheaties cereal as a token of appreciation.

Establish a Problem-Solving Method

Change makers follow specific problem-solving approaches, such as the following:

1. Identify the problem and describe it explicitly, including the effects it has on staff, operations, the bottom line, current and future goals, and patients.

2. Perform a root cause analysis.

3. Generate (or brainstorm) solutions, and weigh the pros and cons of each option.

4. Select the best solution.

5. Develop clear objectives with measures, including timelines and standards.

6. Assign clear roles and responsibilities to those involved in the task.

7. Implement the solution.

8. Monitor progress, making corrections or adjustments along the way if necessary.

9. Communicate with all stakeholders throughout the process.

10. Evaluate the process afterward.

11. Continue to monitor the cause of the problem to ensure no recurrence takes place.

Learn Contemporary Quality-Improvement Concepts

Lean management and Six Sigma are just some of the many tools that leaders can use to improve processes and manage change. Some instruments, such as those developed by the Institute for Healthcare Improvement, are specific to healthcare, but many are adopted from other industries. Change makers stay current about modern improvement techniques and are aware of their advantages, disadvantages, and applications.

Be Willing to Do More

By nature, change makers are always looking for areas to refine, enhance, or study. For some leaders, this improvement could mean increasing the number of their accomplishments for the organization, participating in task forces or forming new ones, or volunteering for new assignments. For others, this could mean expanding their control or creating a new service line. Those who seek added responsibilities or aim for higher achievements may be accused of feeding the needs of their egos. However, the results of this willingness to do more are often beneficial to the organization, yielding enhancements not previously considered.

Network and Benchmark

Change makers are competitive, compelled to compare their results and practices with those of others. They are drawn to data and measurement tools, and they keep abreast of current approaches to forecast future standards. As such, they interact frequently with peers and insiders, visit other sites to scope out new technology and initiatives, and attend conferences and workshops. In sum, these leaders take advantage of any networking opportunity to stay informed, competitive, and innovative.

In contrast, leaders who seldom network and benchmark lose their creative spark and even their perspective. Their strategies and decision making are informed by outdated assumptions.

Learn Change Management

Today, one of the most requested attributes of a leader is the ability to manage and bring about change. Done effectively, change management is a structured process that uses various leadership theories and management models. Although not new, the concept has garnered renewed interest in these times of constant change. Change expert John Kotter (1996; 2002; 2014, 47) enumerates the basic components of change management:

1. Create a sense of urgency.
2. Build a guiding coalition.
3. Form a strategic vision and initiatives.
4. Enlist a volunteer army.
5. Enable action by removing barriers.
6. Generate short-term wins.
7. Sustain acceleration.
8. Institute change.

Change Leadership

In this time of turmoil, healthcare leaders must prioritize change. Kotter International (2011) explains that "change management, which is the term most everyone uses, refers to a set of basic tools or structures intended to keep any change effort under control. The goal is often to minimize the distractions and impacts of the change. Change leadership, on the other hand, concerns the driving forces, visions and processes that fuel large-scale transformation."

Make a Change for Progress's Sake, Not Yours

Some leaders get involved in change efforts because of an inappropriate and selfish need to gain personal fame. They take credit for other people's work and bask in the glory of accomplishment, but they contribute little and pass on the blame if something goes wrong. This behavior does not characterize true change makers.

Change makers pursue change and improvement for the sake of progress, not to strengthen

> The best leaders are those who recognize the situational and follower factors inhibiting or facilitating change, paint a compelling vision of the future, and formulate and execute a plan that moves their vision from a dream to a reality.
>
> —Richard L. Hughes, Robert C. Ginnett, and Gordon J. Curphy (2015)

their power or build up admirers and followers who shower them with adulation and gifts. A health system CEO sums it up well: "In this field, we are entrusted with the lives of people; it is a serious business. And we have to be certain that we make our changes for the betterment of the whole, not just to build our own personal legacies."

CONCLUSION

The leader's value of wanting to make a change is admirable, as it benefits the individual, the organization, and everyone else in between. Change makers strengthen the organization's competitive advantage and reputation, and they help keep out mediocre and stagnant practices and strategies.

Self-Evaluation Questions

❑ What have I accomplished that could be my hallmark of service?

❑ If I were to leave my organization today, how would I be missed? Have I left a "mark" in the organizations in which I've worked?

❑ Flood lines along riverbanks indicate the height the water reached. If I used this parallel to measure my achievement, how high is my flood line?

Case and Exercise
Case 10.1
Kristen Photakis, CEO of a rural hospital, is talking with her friend Jason Weiss, a long-time healthcare consultant, about ways to better engage senior and departmental managers.

KRISTEN. It's frustrating that they sit back and wait for me to create the agenda, give them assignments, or study new trends.

JASON. How does the hospital develop strategies?

KRISTEN. We hold an annual board retreat. During that time, the board and I come up with 25 to 30 goals. When I return to the office, I meet with the vice presidents to tell them what was discussed. Then, I draft subgoals for each of the major objectives identified at the board retreat. The VPs and I hammer out the details until we come up with specific strategies and work plans.

JASON. There are several things wrong with that process. First, everything is developed at the top of the organization with little or no input from the lower ranks. Second, you've gotten into the habit of creating everyone's work plans rather than giving people the chance to develop their own. Third, you and the board set too many goals. You have to consider current workload and priorities, previous commitments, unfinished strategies, et cetera. No one can possibly keep up with all the details. And I must say rather bluntly that you are one of the few organizations I've heard of that does not involve the senior leadership team in the strategic planning retreats with the board. I would make that my starting point.

KRISTEN. Sounds like I have work to do.

JASON. Keep in mind that change is a group effort, not a solo practice. If you want your staff to get involved, you have to get out of the way and let them in.

(continued)

(continued from previous page)

Case 10.1 Questions

1. Is the consultant correct? Explain your answer.

2. What can Kristen do to improve the situation she has created?

Exercise 10.1

The Institute for Healthcare Improvement (IHI; see www.ihi. org) has had a profound impact on change and quality improvement in healthcare. Among IHI's many innovations is rapid-cycle testing, an approach to trying out an idea on a small scale before it is widely implemented. During the testing, the idea is modified if needed and then tried again; the cycle continues until the ideal result is achieved. In the end, the idea is made permanent and applied on a large scale. A key component of rapid-cycle testing is the collection of small sets of data that can be quickly analyzed. These data samples must be carefully picked to ensure that they are representative of the larger data set.

Exercise 10.1 Questions

1. How can rapid-cycle testing improve or harm a leader's ability to make a change?

2. Name other improvement strategies used in the healthcare field today.

REFERENCES

Bolman, L. G, and T. E. Deal. 2013. *Reframing Organizations: Artistry, Choice, and Leadership*, 5th ed. San Francisco: Jossey-Bass.

Dye, C. F., and A. N. Garman. 2015. *Exceptional Leadership: 16 Critical Competencies for Healthcare Leaders*, 2nd ed. Chicago: Health Administration Press.

Forrestal, E. J., and L. W. Cellucci. 2016. *Ethics and Professionalism for Healthcare Managers*. Chicago: Health Administration Press.

Gallup. 2016. "The Culture of an Engaged Workplace: Q12 Engagement." Accessed March 30. www.gallup.com/services/169328/q12-employee-engagement.aspx.

Harter, J., and A. Adkins. 2015. "Employees Want a Lot More from Their Managers." *Gallup Business Journal*. Published April 8. www.gallup.com/businessjournal/182321/employees-lot-managers.aspx.

Haudan, J. 2016. Personal communication with author, May 12.

Hughes, R. L., R. C. Ginnett, and G. J. Curphy. 2015. *Leadership: Enhancing the Lessons of Experience*, 8th ed. Burr Ridge, IL: McGraw-Hill Education.

Isomura, I. 1998. In *Organizational Behavior*, 4th ed., edited by R. Kreiter and A. Kinicki. New York: Richard D. Irwin.

Kotter, J. P. 2014. *Accelerate: Building Strategic Agility for a Faster-Moving World*. Boston: Harvard Business School Press.

———. 2002. *The Heart of Change: Real-Life Stories of How People Change Their Organizations*. Boston: Harvard Business School Press.

———. 1996. *Leading Change*. Boston: Harvard Business School Press.

Kotter International. 2011. "Change Management vs. Change Leadership—What's the Difference?" Published July 12. *Forbes*. www.forbes.com/sites/johnkotter/2011/07/12/change-management-vs-change-leadership-whats-the-difference/#78e0432818ec.

Kouzes, J. M., and B. Z. Posner. 1993. *Credibility: How Leaders Gain and Lose It, Why People Demand It*. San Francisco: Jossey-Bass.

McClelland, D. C. 1961. *The Achieving Society*. New York: Free Press.

Rylatt, A. 2013. "Three Qualities of Highly Successful Change Agents." Association for Talent Development. Published July 8. www.td.org/Publications/Magazines/TD/TD-Archive/2013/07/Three-Qualities-of-Highly-Successful-Change-Agents.

SUGGESTED READING

Haudan, J. 2008. *The Art of Engagement: Bridging the Gap Between People and Possibilities*. New York: McGraw-Hill.

CHAPTER 11

Commitment

*One key to more flow in life comes when we align
what we do with what we enjoy, as is the case with
those fortunate folks whose jobs give them great pleasure.*

—Daniel Goleman (2013)

JUDITH D'AMATO AND Bob Graham, both seasoned vice
presidents at a large medical center, are talking about Blake
Cullen, the newly appointed CEO.

JUDITH. I am amazed at how different she is from the last two
CEOs—Larry Orestes specifically.

BOB. Exactly! Larry practically lived here. He worked more
hours than anyone did and rarely took a vacation. To his
credit, he accomplished a lot. But I can't tell you about a
single project that wasn't contentious or that followed the
initial agreed-on plan. He hated delegating or having others
take the lead. He was exhausting. That's probably why he's
not here anymore.

JUDITH. Blake's energy and focus are admirable. She has a thick
file for every initiative we have rolled out. She asks questions

and pores over material. Despite her packed schedule, she seems to have the time to attend staff events and welcomes people in her office. She's pleasant to be around, and she doesn't intimidate anyone with her skills and high rank.

Bob. Plus, she's so secure with her role that she's not threatened when someone else has better ideas. In fact, she invites and expects us to be part of the process, to do our job. The one thing she strongly demands is that we always keep the mission and vision at the forefront of all our activities.

Judith. It's also clear that she has a life outside of the hospital. Did you know she runs marathons with her grown kids? And every summer, she and her family spend two weeks volunteering to rebuild homes and plant trees in a depressed urban area. One of my nurses told me that. I was inspired.

Bob. That may be one of the major differences between Blake and Larry. She's here because she loves the job and respects the work we do. He was here because he was padding his résumé for the next big move.

EFFECTIVE LEADERSHIP IS a demanding master. It yields not to time. It bends not to excuses. It accepts only commitment.

Commitment is a value that measures the leader's dedication to his profession. Because commitment binds the leader to his work, it generates a strong work ethic, loyalty, pride, productivity, ownership, and even joy.

In exhibit 11.1, several healthcare leaders offer their own definitions of commitment. Some of these definitions use a sports analogy, equating the leader to an athlete and her commitment to an athlete's drive and competitiveness. The primary reason such an analogy is often used is that many leaders view their roles and responsibilities

Exhibit 11.1 Commitment as Defined by Healthcare Executives

- "Getting the job done. You face all the hurdles and finish the race."

- "An attitude of excitement about any problem. Being committed means that you have the chance to fix it."

- "Having a solemn covenant that you will do whatever it takes to fulfill the mission of your organization."

- "The old story of the chicken and the pig. The chicken gave eggs but the pig gave his life. That is true commitment. In some ways, I feel as though I have done the same for the healthcare organizations I have worked for."

- "Giving your all because any race worth running is a race worth winning."

as an athletic event for which they continually train physically, mentally, emotionally, and spiritually.

Great leaders simultaneously act as coaches and players, inspiring and guiding others to do well and performing the work themselves. These leaders are also cheerleaders, boosting morale and applauding efforts. Highly effective leaders do function frequently as coaches, providing guidance, support, and correction. This approach requires a high level of energy and commitment to others. Garman and I describe the competency as mentoring and give specific suggestions on how to mentor (Dye and Garman 2015; see exhibit 11.2).

THE CONCEPT IN PRACTICE

Commitment to the profession is not a given in healthcare, especially in the current environment of high demands but low returns. The following simple strategies help in maintaining commitment.

Exhibit 11.2 How to Mentor

- Understand the career aspirations of your direct reports.

- Work with direct reports to create engaging mentoring plans.

- Support employees in developing their skills.

- Support career development in a nonpossessive way (e.g., know that moving up and moving out are necessary for the career advancement of support staff).

- Find stretch assignments and other delegation opportunities that support skill development.

- Model professional development by advancing your own skills.

Source: Adapted from Dye and Garman (2015).

Stay Focused on the Vision

The organizational vision can serve as a lighthouse and a compass for stewards navigating the choppy waters of healthcare management. It illuminates and points to the path to take. The vision, assuming it was not established arbitrarily and was the result of a careful participative process, takes away the guesswork and indecision about the future state of the organization. Commitment to the cause, so to speak, is easier with this desired outcome in full view. Great leaders prefer to know where they are going before they even start the journey.

Weigh Work and Life Pursuits

In recent years, the option to work from home has become a sought-after benefit for many workers. Many leaders and managers, however, have been exercising this capability for as long as reports and deadlines have been around. Smartphones, tablets, and laptops have exacerbated this practice, equipping leaders to work before and after business hours and even during vacations. In the twenty-first century, everyone (even those in nonmanagement positions) seems to be overworked, running ragged to keep up with heavy workloads and short turnarounds.

Unfortunately, leaders who are constantly working lose perspective and burn out. They place excessive demands on their staff and have unreasonable expectations. As a result, workplace morale becomes low; many mistakes are made; distrust spreads; productivity suffers; and employees become stressed out, fearful, and difficult to retain and manage. Employees do not even get a respite when overworked bosses are away from the office, as these leaders check in by e-mail or phone.

> The ultimate test of a servant leader's work is whether those served develop toward being more responsible, caring, and competent individuals.
>
> —Richard L. Hughes, Robert C. Ginnett, and Gordon J. Curphy (2015)

Another, and most important, casualty of overworking is the executive's personal life. For every high achiever, there is a patient and supportive family member (e.g., spouse, partner, parent, child) who has been overlooked or a personal pursuit (e.g., hobby, advanced degree, creative aspiration, spiritual development) that has been pushed aside. Over the long run, this situation could result in resentment at best and family and social breakdown at worst.

A new school of thought argues that maintaining a work–life balance has become a fallacy in a deadline- and travel-intensive global market. What matters, according to this theory, is the flexibility to respond to both work and life demands and an awareness of the consequences when one is chosen over another. In this sense, work and life are integrated, not separate entities that do not meet. That said, leaders should learn ways to cope with the demands of both work and life with the goal of doing their best at these two components. Exhibit 11.3 offers strategies for maintaining career success without sacrificing personal interests.

Find an Enjoyable Outlet

Healthcare pushes many of its executives to the limit. Many leaders are fatigued and tapped out and want to change careers.

Exhibit 11.3 How to Maintain Both Work and Life Pursuits

Minimize meetings. Many meetings are often unnecessary. Before you attend or host one, ask the following questions:

- What is the goal of this meeting?
- Can this goal be achieved without my presence?
- Can this goal be accomplished through other means, including e-mail exchanges or memos?
- What other work could I do if I do not attend this meeting?
- Could I delegate attendance at this meeting to someone else?

Prioritize work and life to-dos. First, write two comprehensive lists—one for work responsibilities, one for personal priorities. Second, categorize items on both lists as urgent (U), important (I), or can wait (CW). Third, assign an order to the items in each category (1 for first to be done, 2 for next, etc.) according to level of importance. Such a priority list serves as a visual reminder and a stress reducer because the items are part of your daily functions, not just weighing on your mind.

Allow for regular downtime. Schedule a block of time every week, for at least two to three hours, to get away from job stressors. Even if you cannot physically leave the workplace and stop all tasks, take time out to tend to low-pressure activities. Some executives take one or two days away from the office every couple of months to regroup. Unplugging from wireless devices or smartphones for at least several hours a day is also a wise move.

Be flexible with time. A tight schedule does not allow for the surprises inherent in healthcare operations. The same is true for personal life. Being flexible does not mean ignoring the calendar altogether, but it does mean having a willingness to accommodate unplanned or unforeseen demands, whether they are work related or home related.

Get regular exercise. Regular physical activity boosts energy levels and helps clear the mind.

Volunteer. Giving back to the community not only improves your reputation but also gives you fresh perspectives. Join the board of a local service organization, participate in fund-raising activities, or perform outreach work for a cause you would like to advance. Volunteering is an ideal activity in which to involve your friends and family.

An undertaking that has nothing to do with the field can refresh a leader who is suffering from burnout. It presents opportunities for developing out-of-the-box solutions and stimulates thinking. It also hones teamwork and learning skills, as well as the leader's humility, as she is now a follower instead of the main person in charge.

Simply spending time with family and friends can be an enjoyable outlet.

Show Initiative

The greatest proof of a leader's commitment is her initiative. Initiative is the drive to chart a new direction with no outside encouragement or command. Some healthcare leaders define initiative as follows:

- "Doing more than is required—going the extra mile."
- "Actively seeking out issues and problems."
- "Being proactive, not reactive."
- "Engaging in positive thinking."
- "Not being a minimalist."
- "Avoiding the negativity of blaming others and acting like a victim of circumstances."

Only by taking the initiative can you follow your own course. As the Spanish poet Antonio Machado (2003, 239) writes, "Traveler, there is no road. . . . As you walk, you make your own road."

Be Prepared to Make Sacrifices

Leadership expert John C. Maxwell (2007, 198) says, "Sacrifice is a constant in leadership. It is an ongoing process, not a one-time payment." The advice "you must pay your dues" is often given

> Subordinates often become committed to goals simply by seeing the sincere and enthusiastic commitment of top leadership to them.
>
> — Richard L. Hughes, Robert C. Ginnett, and Gordon J. Curphy (2015)

in healthcare, which is primarily hierarchical in structure. As such, the expectation is that those interested in moving up the organizational ladder need to yield to the demands (and politics) of their positions, investing much energy and time in their projects and performing work that no one else opts to do. For example, new health administration program graduates are assigned tasks, such as copying and cold calling, that do not require an advanced degree. Similarly, middle managers are sent out to attend time-consuming, low-level meetings or to handle face-to-face patient complaints. The purpose of these seemingly menial assignments is not to punish the employees but to test their team orientation, "get-to-it-tiveness," and commitment to their careers.

Making sacrifices, however, is not confined to non–senior management staff. Executives are also expected to make concessions for the good of the enterprise or the team. Over time, such sacrifices build up, giving the executive a bank of goodwill that can be drawn on when needed.

In a way, making sacrifices is an American value because it is based on the principle of "hard work merits rewards." The American public generally scoffs at people who rely on their good fortune, not years of honest effort and even failure, to become successful.

Think Positively

Positive thinking is a deliberate act, a choice that can be made in the face of negative scenarios. It transforms bad attitudes and victim mentalities, and it overtakes people's tendency to fear the worst. Committed leaders make a conscious decision to think positively and have a good attitude because they want their initiatives to succeed. Even when an effort is, by all indications, going to have less-than-optimal outcomes, committed leaders dwell on the bright side—that is, they look for lessons, instead of mistakes. Mistakes have a negative connotation that makes people wary and defensive. Lessons, on the other hand, focus on improvement and development.

Positive thinking has its share of detractors who contend that it shields us from reality and thus sets us up for disappointment. This pessimistic view, however, may breed bad attitudes that only perpetuate the difficulty of any situation and weaken commitment. Perhaps a more relevant possibility to consider is the one proposed by Collinson (2012, 87), who suggests that "leaders' excessive positivity is often characterized by a reluctance to consider alternative voices, which can leave organizations and societies ill-prepared to deal with unexpected events." He continues to argue that this type of leadership "encourages leaders to believe their own narratives that everything is going well and discourages followers from raising problems or admitting mistakes" (87). However, Mohanty (2014, 61) presents the counterargument: "The leader's attitude tends to spread and affect others drastically. A good leader truly cares about the morale of the team [and] motivates his team with respect [and] a relentlessly positive attitude. The success of any organization is very much dependent on the leadership attitude. The role of a leader is to inspire people so that they can contribute their best to the organization and also inspire them to become more confident in their work to achieve their personal and group goals, [which] reflects the attitude of a leader."

Exhibit 11.4 provides Gandhi's insight into the power of a positive spirit and its impact on literally all that you will do.

Be Mindful of Body Language

A leader's body language and facial cues communicate many messages. For example, a leader's frown as he paces the hallway could signal stress, while his warm smile and leisurely walk may represent his approachability. Commitment (or lack thereof) can be displayed through body language as well. Uncrossed arms, eye contact, leaning slightly into the other person, and standing or sitting to be equal in height with that person are just some examples.

Exhibit 11.4 Positive Attitudes: From Your Thoughts to Your Destiny

Keep your thoughts positive, because your thoughts become your words.

Keep your words positive, because your words become your behavior.

Keep your behavior positive, because your behavior becomes your habits.

Keep your habits positive, because your habits become your values.

Keep your values positive, because your values become your destiny.

—Mahatma Gandhi

Source: Reprinted from Gold (2002).

Promote Employee Participation and Engagement

As discussed in chapter 10, ensuring staff satisfaction is no longer enough; leaders must also encourage employees to take part in organizational efforts. One way to support engagement is to delegate responsibility to staff.

Many healthcare workers, including managers, are highly reliable and intelligent. They await an opportunity from their superiors to use their skills and judgment on an important initiative. Such an assignment contributes to the employee's sense of commitment to her job and to the organization, not to mention to the processes and outcomes of the project or task.

> The more one's authority and breadth of responsibilities increase, the more control there should be over one's own time and commitments.
>
> —Ted W. Engstrom and Edward R. Dayton (1984)

This manager–worker connection could inspire other involvement, including that of physicians, patients, and families. Employee engagement could increase morale and help in the recruitment and retention of high performers. Exhibit 11.5 enumerates the contributors to employee engagement.

Exhibit 11.5 Organizational Factors That Contribute to Employee Engagement

Excellent organizational reputation. Highly engaged employees are found in organizations known for providing high-quality care and other public services to their community.

Clear job expectations. Highly engaged employees know exactly what their roles, responsibilities, and goals are.

Close relationships with supervisors. Highly engaged employees report to managers who leverage the staff's individual capabilities and meet their professional needs.

Regular feedback. Highly engaged employees receive frequent comments on their individual and team performance for the purpose of learning and improvement.

Recognition and celebration. Highly engaged employees appreciate rewards and celebrations for their efforts.

Career advancement and continuous education. Highly engaged employees are encouraged to pursue educational interests and in-house promotional opportunities.

Develop a Strong System of Personal Organization

Being organized is a symbol of being committed. It signals that the leader is always in control of her time, tasks, and priorities, among other things. Such a leader uses all available tools, such as filing systems, calendars or planners, and smartphones. A personal assistant helps the leader manage her schedule.

CONCLUSION

To committed leaders, work is not drudgery or toil; instead, it offers great satisfaction. In the classic book *The 7 Habits of Highly Effective*

People, Stephen Covey (2013) lists being proactive as the first habit. According to Covey, being proactive is a function of commitment and work ethic. Now, imagine an organization teeming with proactive workers and leaders, then realize that your organization can become one, too. As the saying goes, "Practice makes perfect."

Self-Evaluation Questions

❑ What does commitment mean to me?

❑ Am I paying a price for the work I do? Is that price worth the rewards I am receiving? Do I enjoy my work?

❑ What does "paying dues" mean to me?

❑ If my staff were to describe my facial expressions at work, what would they say?

❑ To what degree am I organized? Do I regularly run behind schedule? Do I keep a daily or weekly to-do list and accomplish most, if not all, of it?

❑ Consider this quote from Katzenbach and Smith (1993, 105): "Team [members] work hard and enthusiastically. They also play hard and enthusiastically. No one has to ask them to put in extra time; they just do it. No one has to remind them not to delegate jobs to others; again, they just do the work themselves. To outsiders, the energy and enthusiasm levels inside teams are unmistakable and even seductive." To what extent does this description apply to my contributions to the team?

Case and Exercises
Case 11.1
Children's Hospital has a reputation for having the lowest turnover rate among the six hospitals located in the area,

despite the fact that its average wages are approximately 10 percent lower than those offered by its competitors. In addition, Children's Hospital has the highest rate of employee engagement. In contrast, University Hospital, which provides the largest compensation and benefit packages in the area, has the highest rate of turnover and the lowest rate of employee engagement.

Dori Shimbuku, a human resources consultant hired by University Hospital to study its recruitment and retention patterns, comes to the conclusion that University employees, including its leaders and managers, lack commitment.

Case 11.1 Questions
1. What does Dori mean? What should she recommend University Hospital do to increase employee and leadership commitment?

2. How might commitment be measured?

Exercise 11.1
Several online articles discuss employee engagement. Choose two of them and develop a presentation that answers the following questions:

1. What are the primary causes of high employee engagement?

2. What is the relationship between an employee's level of engagement and his relationship with his boss?

3. What practices should senior leaders develop to build employee engagement in their organizations?

The online resources on Employee Engagement included at the end of this chapter may be useful for this exercise.

(continued)

(continued from previous page)

Exercise 11.2
Physician engagement has become a widely discussed topic. Conduct an online search for information about physician engagement, and determine the applicability of the concept of commitment to enhancing physician engagement.

REFERENCES

Collinson, D. 2012. "Prozac Leadership and the Limits of Positive Thinking." *Leadership* 8 (2): 87–107.

Covey, S. R. 2013. *The 7 Habits of Highly Successful People: Powerful Lessons in Personal Change*, 25th anniversary ed. New York: Simon and Schuster.

Dye, C. F., and A. N. Garman. 2015. *Exceptional Leadership: 16 Critical Competencies for Healthcare Leaders*, 2nd ed. Chicago: Health Administration Press.

Engstrom, T. W., and E. R. Dayton. 1984. *The Christian Leader's 60-Second Management Guide*. Waco, TX: Word Books.

Gold, T. 2002. *Open Your Mind, Open Your Life: A Little Book of Eastern Wisdom*. Kansas City, MO: Andrews McMeel Publishing.

Goleman, D. 2013. *Focus: The Hidden Driver of Excellence*. New York: HarperCollins.

Hughes, R. L., R. C. Ginnett, and G. J. Curphy. 2015. *Leadership: Enhancing the Lessons of Experience*, 8th ed. Burr Ridge, IL: McGraw-Hill Education.

Katzenbach, J. R., and D. K. Smith. 1993. *The Wisdom of Teams: Creating the High-Performance Organization*. Boston: Harvard Business Press.

Machado, A. 2003. *There Is No Road*. Translated by M. C. Berg and D. Maloney. Buffalo, NY: White Pine Press.

Maxwell, J. C. 2007. *Ultimate Leadership: Maximize Your Potential and Empower Your Team*. Nashville, TN: Thomas Nelson.

Mohanty, S. 2014. "A Leader with Positive Attitude and Thinking Can Bring Great Success." *International Journal of Emerging Research in Management and Technology* 3 (2): 61–63.

SUGGESTED READINGS

Collinson, D., and D. Tourish. 2015. "Teaching Leadership Critically: New Directions for Leadership Pedagogy." *Academy of Management Learning and Education* 14 (4): 576–94.

Cunha, M. P., A. Rego, S. Clegg, and P. Neves. 2013. "The Case for Transcendent Followership." *Leadership* 9 (1): 87–106.

Lewis, K. R. 2015. "Everything You Need to Know About Your Millennial Coworkers." *Fortune*. Published June 23. http://fortune.com/2015/06/23/know-your-millennial-co-workers/.

Turkel, M. C., G. Reidinger, K. Ferket, and K. Reno. 2005. "An Essential Component of the Magnet Journey: Fostering an Environment for Evidence-Based Practice and Nursing Research." *Nursing Administration Quarterly* 29 (3): 254–62.

Yahaya, R., and F. Ebrahim. 2016. "Leadership Styles and Organizational Commitment: Literature Review." *Journal of Management Development* 35 (2): 190–216.

Zhang, X., N. Li, J. Ullrich, and R. van Dick. 2015. "Getting Everyone on Board: The Effect of Differentiated Transformational Leadership by CEOs on Top Management Team Effectiveness and Leader-Rated Firm Performance." *Journal of Management* 41 (7): 1898–933.

ONLINE RESOURCES ON EMPLOYEE ENGAGEMENT

Dale Carnegie Training. 2012. "What Drives Employee Engagement and Why It Matters." Accessed May 18, 2016. www.dale carnegie.com/assets/1/7/driveengagement_101612_wp.pdf.

Gallup. 2016a. "The Culture of an Engaged Workplace: Q12 Engagement." Accessed March 30. www.gallup.com/services/169328/q12-employee-engagement.aspx.

————. 2016b. "Employee Engagement." Accessed May 18. www.gallup.com/topic/employee_engagement.aspx.

Graber, S. 2015. "The Two Sides of Employee Engagement." *Harvard Business Review*. Published December 4. https://hbr.org/2015/12/the-two-sides-of-employee-engagement.

Harter, J., and A. Adkins. 2015. "What Great Managers Do to Engage Their Employees." *Harvard Business Review*. Published April 2. https://hbr.org/2015/04/what-great-managers-do-to-engage-employees.

Ryan, L. 2015. "What Does 'Employee Engagement' Mean?" *Forbes*. Published April 4. www.forbes.com/sites/lizryan/2015/04/04/what-does-employee-engagement-mean/#19cd2a729ab3.

CHAPTER 12

Emotional Intelligence

No matter what leaders set out to do—
whether it's creating strategy or mobilizing teams
to action—their success depends on how *they do it.*

—Daniel Goleman, Richard Boyatzis,
and Annie McKee (2013)

DURING LUNCH AT an off-site leadership seminar, a group of middle managers from the same health system participates in an open dialogue about the vice presidents in their various hospitals.

KYLA. The strongest of the group is Melissa Varga. Her departments meet budgets year in and year out. Their clinical outcomes are high, and their retention is great. I'd like to work for that vice president.

ANDREW. Well, I do work for her and I wish I didn't. Melissa is an emotional roller coaster. Some days she is calm, and some days she just seems crazed. Behind closed doors, she is not beyond using threats to get us to achieve our goals, but often all that outsiders see is this calm and controlled leader. She's far from that. We're expected to work many hours, and she's always frowning when we take vacation. My business units are all work and no play. We're really stuck with her because she has all the clinical departments reporting to her.

BJ. I heard she throws tantrums. I was going to apply for a job working for her, but someone warned me. I'm glad to work for Mike Randolph. This guy is one cool cucumber. He constantly gets things done and does not get overexcited when things go wrong. He expresses thanks to us and respects our work, so we respect him back. He has very good interpersonal skills and controls his emotions. Even under pressure, he doesn't lose his composure.

KYLA. He sounds like a robot, but better than Melissa, it seems. What's the difference then—they actually both achieve high results?

ANDREW. Both of them are pretty strong execs. I think the difference is emotional intelligence.

BJ. Well, that's just a catchall phrase without much meaning. What is it, really?

KYLA. It means the person has a good grasp of his or her emotions and feelings and how those are displayed externally. Leadership is not exclusively about getting results. It's getting results without emotional outbursts or allowing anger to take over. Actually, I think there's some pretty good research that shows that emotional intelligence is a legitimate thing.

IN THE LATE 1990s, writer Daniel Goleman popularized the concept of emotional intelligence, setting off further inquiries into the relationship between feelings and intellect. Researchers Peter Salovey and Jack Mayer (1990, 189), two pioneers of emotional intelligence, define the term as follows: "Emotional intelligence [is] the subset of social intelligence that involves the ability to monitor one's own and others' feelings and emotions, to discriminate among them and to use this information to guide one's thinking and actions."

Emotional intelligence has two components: energy and maturity. Energy (or the spark or zeal for life) refers to the liveliness and stamina with which people approach their work. It keeps leaders fresh and motivated when others have had enough and are ready to give up. Maturity, meanwhile, refers to people's refinement, social graces, tact, capacity to grow and change, and ability to interpret signals from others. It makes leaders aware of signals from others. It reminds leaders to apologize, express gratitude, harbor no ill will, empathize, have a sense of humor, and respect others. Also, maturity keeps leaders poised during times of distress and wise during times of pressure. Although maturity is often associated with old age, it can be learned at a young age.

Emotionally intelligent leaders make every effort to develop their leadership skills, knowledge, and abilities. They also work hard to be aware of their inner emotional selves and the world around them. They are confident and enthusiastic and have self-esteem and a positive attitude. They discern nuances in (and thus are sensitive to) people's words and actions. They are aware of the effect that their (and others') needs, beliefs, motivations, and feelings have on their surroundings. They know how damaging passive-aggressive behaviors and one-upmanship can be in the workplace. They are watchful of situations in which they and others deal with conflict, criticisms, stress, pressure, and difficult people. They use a self-awareness lens, which enables them to see the communication and behavioral patterns that showcase the worst in people, including themselves.

Simply put, emotionally intelligent leaders have a robust capability for reading people and receiving and giving critical feedback. This ability comes

> Your first and foremost job as a leader is to take charge of your own energy and then to orchestrate the energy of those around you.
>
> —Peter Drucker (quoted in Mycek 1997)

from their firm understanding of their own and others' feelings and the environment in which they operate.

THE SELF-AWARENESS FACTOR

In the book *Emotional Intelligence at Work*, author Hendrie Weisinger (1998) sets out the following steps to improving emotional intelligence:

1. Develop high self-esteem.
2. Manage your emotions.
3. Motivate yourself.
4. Develop effective command skills.
5. Develop interpersonal expertise.
6. Help others help themselves.

According to Weisinger, self-awareness is the main driver of these steps. Self-awareness is a universal panacea for negativity and enables leaders to

- accept (even anticipate) constructive criticism;
- avoid feeling defensive;
- support those around them;
- be assertive but not aggressive;
- have confidence in their ability to initiate change;
- view scenarios as win–win;
- not be hostile, overbearing, or impatient; and
- take charge of situations.

Conversely, leaders who are not self-aware misinterpret events and others' comments, throw tantrums or act out, and are reactive rather than proactive.

Many executives, because of their high rank, have become so removed from daily operations and workers that they do not even realize how others in the organization perceive them. When in the office, they primarily deal with their direct reports, a group that mainly consists of other senior managers who are likely also isolated from staff. As a result, these executives' workplace reality becomes distorted and their emotional intelligence dulls.

Worse, their self-awareness is based on incomplete information or incorrect assumptions about themselves and others.

THE CONCEPT IN PRACTICE

The following principles can enhance emotional intelligence.

Develop Personal and Social Competence

Experts suggest that emotional intelligence may be managed through learning and improving both personal and social competencies. Personal competency includes self-awareness, self-control, and self-motivation. Social competency, meanwhile, includes social awareness, empathy, collaboration, and teamwork. According to Singh (2010, 41), "An attempt to develop the personal competencies of executives in [an] organization can go a long way to improve their emotional intelligence."

Characteristics of Emotionally Intelligent Leaders

Comfortable and self-aware. They are confident with their skills, goals, and visions but value continuous improvement. Thus, they welcome feedback.

Reflective listener. They show a genuine interest in other people and their ideas. They encourage others to lead discussions or give input. They rarely interrupt, preferring instead to wait their turn.

Nonthreatening and nonintimidating. They are open and approachable. They do not use power to manipulate their followers, and they are aware that the trappings of their high rank are easily misunderstood and could corrupt their reputation.

Available. They avoid appearing constantly busy, as it signals that they do not highly regard the everyday tasks and challenges of employees. They invite others to speak with them directly, and they attend events of great importance to staff.

Seek Feedback

Emotionally intelligent leaders do not feel threatened by feedback, whether from direct discussions or through 360-degree assessment tools. These executives relish the chance to receive ratings and comments from peers, subordinates, and other associates because they understand the role of feedback in their personal and professional development.

Appendix B presents the Emotional Intelligence Evaluation Form, a tool that leaders can use to obtain direct feedback. This instrument works best when there is participation from staff and associates at all levels of the organization so that a comprehensive result can be generated. To ensure the confidentiality of the feedback, participants are discouraged from sharing their comments. Ideally, a neutral third party should administer the tool, collate comments, and provide a full report to the leader being evaluated.

Set a Personal Path and Follow It

Many individuals—leaders included—possess little sense of personal direction, especially when they get caught up in the busyness of daily operations. These leaders may be effective in establishing and monitoring organizational objectives, but they may fall short when managing their own careers.

Emotionally intelligent leaders, in contrast, frequently take stock of where they have been and what they have accomplished. They know their long-term and short-term personal goals and seek to work in organizations that provide opportunities for fulfilling those goals. In other words, they look for fit between their personal mission and the organization's mission so that both entities can benefit from the union. For example, an individual who intends to make a difference in the public health system is not served well by working in a large for-profit.

Some emotionally intelligent leaders weigh their career options by occasionally interviewing for open positions even when they do not intend to leave their jobs. This exercise allows them to compare their skills and accomplishments with current standards and expectations.

Leaders who are not attuned to their personal intentions or path can more easily get derailed by the unceasing demands of healthcare management.

View Annual Retreats as a Time for Self-Reflection

Most members of religious orders and some laypersons often take religious retreats. These are planned getaways, lasting a few days to a week, that focus on intense introspection. Although these retreats are intended to reconnect participants with their original aspirations, some people go a step further: They reflect on their own strengths and weaknesses and incorporate their abilities into their leadership style. One nun admits to designing a succession plan while on a retreat.

Get a Coach

Executive or leadership coaching has become one of the fastest-growing areas of consulting, as leaders have realized the benefits of having a neutral adviser. These coaches can assess current behavior, management style, and performance; offer unbiased feedback; and teach practical skills for improvement and for managing perceptions. In addition, coaches are helpful in establishing a clear career vision or direction. Large numbers of physician leaders, in particular, use leadership coaches. Winters (2013) reports that they "feel under-qualified to lead," so they seek coaches to understand leadership and emotional intelligence issues more keenly.

Many emotionally intelligent leaders rely on their coaches, with whom they discuss private details of their jobs and from whom they seek counsel. The book *Exceptional Leadership* (Dye and Garman 2015, 195–203) presents an entire chapter on how to use executive coaches. Several coaching websites also offer information on this topic—see, for example, www.theexecutivecoachingforum.com and www.coachnet.com.

Manage Your Emotions

Managing emotions is not the same as lacking emotions. In this era of social media—when sharing personal information, opinions, and reactions has become routine practice for anyone with an account—it is easy to assume that those who maintain composure have no feelings or are "robots." Emotionally intelligent people do, in fact, have a lot of emotions—only they tend to show more positive feelings (e.g., optimism, sympathy, confidence), rather than negative ones (e.g., defeat, anger, vengeance). Most important, they *manage* their emotions.

Emotionally intelligent leaders know that positive messages are influential, inspiring followers and keeping them enthused about initiatives, even the difficult ones. Negative emotions, on the other hand, are not motivational. They instill fear and anxiety, and they could erode trust and respect.

Executives do reach points at which their frustrations take over—a natural occurrence in management. Over time, these emotional outbursts could devolve into an angry personality that the person is not able to discern in himself. Cursing, shouting, name-calling, chronic complaining, and impatience are some signs of poor emotional control. Weisinger (1998) notes that physiological changes can be observed in people who "lose their cool," including heart palpitations, perspiration, and rapid respiration.

Although emotions are a natural response to everyday stimuli, they can become detrimental in

> Emotional competence is particularly central to leadership. . . . Interpersonal ineptitude in leaders lowers everyone's performance: It wastes time, creates acrimony, corrodes motivation and commitment, builds hostility and apathy.
>
> —Daniel Goleman (1998)

the workplace if they are not appropriately displayed. Leaders should watch out for their personal emotional triggers (and the responses described by Weisinger) in an effort to slow down or transform their reactions.

Expect Setbacks

Leaders respond to setbacks differently. Because they are more optimistic, emotionally intelligent leaders cope well with challenges. Some of these leaders take a mental or physical break from the activity and return with renewed commitment, while others view setbacks as a personal test they must pass. To better deal with setbacks, one CEO carries around a laminated card with the following message:

> You will get knocked down at times.
> You will taste dirt occasionally.
> But it is through this process that
> You will better enjoy the return to the air above.

Maintain Physical and Mental Health

Healthcare delivery is physically and mentally exhausting work, even for those who do not provide direct care. As such, healthcare leaders must maintain their health, which enables them to be of service to their staff and patients. Appropriate amounts of rest, sleep, and exercise and a balanced diet go a long way toward wellness. A regular visit to the doctor, vacations or time off, and a stress-decreasing routine also help.

The point is that leaders who are too tired or too physically and mentally rundown are ineffective, negative, and short-tempered. They are not approachable, and they behave unpredictably, to the detriment of the employees and the organization. Emotional intelligence cannot be developed and sustained in an unhealthy mind and body.

View Everything Holistically

Highly effective leaders know that life has ups and downs, and that, as leaders, they will likely have more ups and downs than other workers do. Maintaining perspective and seeing the whole picture, however, helps them manage emotions. Exhibit 12.1 shows how this flows.

CONCLUSION

Emotional intelligence is more critical today given that the command-and-control style of leadership is no longer the norm. More and more leaders understand that they have to earn—not expect—respect and trust. Being emotionally intelligent is one way to practice this understanding. Emotionally intelligent leaders do not use their power to gain an advantage over others; are aware of their intentions, accomplishments, and shortcomings; manage their emotions; and welcome feedback. This level of maturity requires a lot of work, something that an emotionally intelligent leader puts in every day.

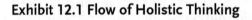

Exhibit 12.1 Flow of Holistic Thinking

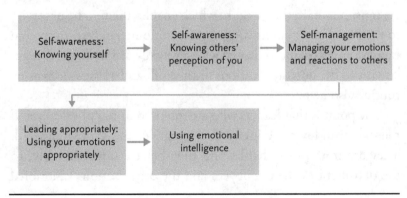

Self-Evaluation Questions

☐ How isolated have I become from direct personal feedback?

☐ How well do I know myself?

☐ Would others say that I am plagued by frequent bouts of emotional inconsistency, such as outbursts of anger, hostility, or antagonism?

☐ How do I manage my emotions?

Case and Exercise

Case 12.1

Mike Sebastian has been the director of facilities for more than 30 years. Up until the past three years, the facilities department had low turnover. Today, however, the turnover rate is 30 percent, causing concern for Rena Shah, the chief human resources officer at the hospital.

To understand the problem, Rena pays a visit to several of Mike's former employees.

FIRST WORKER. I retired because of him. I couldn't take the constant panic he gave me. He wasn't that bad when he first started—a little temperamental but nothing to complain about. But he changed a lot in my last years there. He would blow his top when he found out something was not done or someone made a complaint about us. It was hard to live with.

SECOND WORKER. I quit six months after he hired me. Mike was a screamer. People outside the department didn't know because he seemed great with everyone

(continued)

(continued from previous page)

else. Behind closed doors, though, he could dress you down. No job was worth that. Even though I needed the money and was really looking forward to being eligible for the pension plan, I decided to leave for my own peace of mind.

THIRD WORKER. Forget about talking to him! He would never listen. He's old school. He thinks it's his way or the highway. I once tried to reason with him to calm down the situation, but he fired me. And I put in the best years of my life in that job. With all due respect, Ms. Shah, you should give him the boot and give him a taste of his own medicine.

Case 12.1 Questions
1. How should Rena address the problem with Mike?
2. What do you think triggered Mike's transformation in the past three years?

Exercise 12.1
As mentioned earlier, emotional intelligence may be managed through learning and improving both personal and social competencies. Personal competency includes self-awareness, self-control, and self-motivation. Social competency, meanwhile, includes social awareness, empathy, collaboration, and teamwork.

Go to the website of Consortium for Research on Emotional Intelligence in Organizations (www.eiconsortium.org) and develop a list of the specific leadership behaviors that characterize emotional intelligence. How do these behaviors match up with your own?

REFERENCES

Dye, C. F., and A. N. Garman. 2015. *Exceptional Leadership: 16 Critical Competencies for Healthcare Executives*, 2nd ed. Chicago: Health Administration Press.

Goleman, D. 1998. *Working with Emotional Intelligence*. New York: Bantam Books.

Goleman, D., R. Boyatzis, and A. McKee. 2013. *Primal Leadership: Unleashing the Power of Emotional Intelligence*. Boston: Harvard Business Review Press.

Mycek, S. 1997. "Getting Beyond Industrial Logic: Renewing Our Faith in the Value of Health." *Healthcare Forum Journal* 40 (4): 16–20.

Salovey, P., and J. D. Mayer. 1990. "Emotional Intelligence." *Imagination, Cognition, and Personality* 9 (3): 185–211.

Singh, K. 2010. "Developing Human Capital by Linking Emotional Intelligence with Personal Competencies in Indian Business Organizations." *International Journal of Business Science and Applied Management* 5 (2): 29–42.

Weisinger, H. 1998. *Emotional Intelligence at Work: The Untapped Edge for Success*. San Francisco: Jossey-Bass.

Winters, R. 2013. "Coaching Physicians to Become Leaders." *Harvard Business Review*. Published October 7. https://hbr.org/2013/10/coaching-physicians-to-become-leaders/.

SUGGESTED READINGS

Boak, G. 2016. "Enabling Team Learning in Healthcare." *Action Learning: Research and Practice* 13 (2): 101–17.

Jafri, M. H., C. Dem, and S. Choden. 2016. "Emotional Intelligence and Employee Creativity: Moderating Role of Proactive Personality and Organizational Climate." *Business Perspectives and Research* 4 (1): 54–66.

Schlaerth, A., N. Ensari, and J. Christian. 2013. "A Meta-analytical Review of the Relationship Between Emotional Intelligence and Leaders' Constructive Conflict Management." *Group Processes and Intergroup Relations* 16 (1): 126–36.

Spano-Szekely, L., M. T. Quinn Griffin, J. Clavelle, and J. J. Fitzpatrick. "Emotional Intelligence and Transformational Leadership in Nurse Managers." *Journal of Nursing Administration* 46 (2): 101–18.

Thompson, J. A., and R. Fairchild. 2013. "Does Nurse Manager Education Really Matter?" *Nursing Management* 44 (9): 10–14.

Tyczkowski, B., C. Vandenhouten, J. Reilly, G. Bansal, S. M. Kubsch, and R. Jakkola. 2015. "Emotional Intelligence (EI) and Nursing Leadership Styles Among Nurse Managers." *Nursing Administration Quarterly* 39 (2): 172–80.

Ungaretti, T., K. R. Thompson, A. Miller, and T. O. Peterson. 2015. "Problem-Based Learning: Lessons from Medical Education and Challenges for Management Education." *Academy of Management Learning* 14 (2): 173–86.

PART III

TEAM VALUES

CHAPTER 13

Cooperation and Sharing

The reliance on teams is due partially to increasingly complex tasks, more globalization, and the flattening of organizational structure.

—Peter G. Northouse (2016)

THE PROFESSOR OPENS his class with a question: "As you know, I do a lot of executive team building and executive coaching with senior leaders across the country. What do you think is the greatest challenge in getting senior executives to work together in a collaborative and cooperative way?"

His students volunteer the following responses:

- Most of them don't have the time to be part of a good team.
- A lot of their work takes place outside the team with other teams and groups of people. They really aren't together that much.
- Executives do not fit well into teams. They are pretty arrogant, probably don't play well in the sandbox together, and have to follow what the CEO says. I just don't see them as team players.

- At that level, there's more interest in who gets the credit for the job.
- They're not really all equals. Probably the chief financial officer or the chief nursing officer or someone like that is really viewed at a higher level than the others. Without equality, you can't get a team to work.

The professor replies, "Those are all good thoughts! The real challenge, from what I have experienced, has been participation—that is, active participation. If all the team members participate, then I can help them build an atmosphere of sharing. That's when the team becomes focused on shared goals and mutual trust."

TOO MANY MEETINGS today have a hypnotizing show-and-tell style: One by one, meeting attendees tell the others about their project and show (with PowerPoints and handouts) how the project is progressing. Questions and answers are volleyed, but often very little attention is given to identifying the problems that could arise, or have arisen, from the undertaking. No one asks about the details of or the reasons for the project, and few volunteer their help. And there is always the "sneak peek" at e-mails or texts. At the end of these meetings, people file out no more involved with others' projects. Consequently, when successes or failures happen, they become an individual's accomplishment or failure, rather than a team's celebration or setback.

Although the healthcare field prides itself on emphasizing individual authority and accountability (especially in a physician clinical environment), it should also support and encourage team dynamics. Building teams means encouraging efficiencies.

Teams are predestined for failure when they lack the fundamental values of teamwork: cooperation and sharing. Both elements require team members' willingness and the team leader's encouragement and support. Simply put, cooperation and sharing demand that team members sacrifice some of their individuality for the benefit of the entire team.

THE CONCEPT IN PRACTICE

Strengthen your team with the following strategies.

Build the Right Team from the Start

Most CEOs who come into an organization rebuild all or at least part of their executive team. They do this for two reasons: (1) to establish their mark on the organization and (2) to assemble a team of people who espouse similar values. Most executives who are tapped to become part of the new team are excited about the opportunity. Often, this excitement translates to wanting to share and cooperate.

When recruiting, leaders must consider people who believe in the concept of teams. They should evaluate prospective members with the following guidelines:

1. Ask prospects to recount an actual situation in which they worked with a team and by doing so developed a solution

Team effort enhances . . .

Coordination, reducing bureaucracy. Assigning specific functions to people helps eliminate overlapping responsibilities, duplication of duties, and red tape.

Involvement and support. Because everyone works together toward a common goal, the focus shifts from receiving personal glory and recognition to supporting the team's objectives and valuing the contributions of others. "That's not my job" is replaced by "It's everybody's job."

General oversight, reducing problems that fall through the cracks. Everyone is involved in making sure that nothing is overlooked or undermined.

The joy of celebrations. One of the reasons sports bind people together is that everyone enjoys watching the exhilaration of team victories. An accomplishment is always grander when more people share and enjoy it because it represents the combination of each person's hard work, sacrifice, and dedication.

Creativity. When more people are involved, various perspectives and new ideas are generated and better results are achieved.

that was much better than their own. Listen carefully for the candidate's behavior and their inclination—or disinclination—toward teamwork.

2. Ask prospects to recount an actual situation in which they had problems working with teams. Ask them how they handled their frustration.

3. Ask prospects to describe a situation in which team efforts do not work very well.

4. Ask prospects to name the values that drive effective team interaction (see chapter 17).

5. Administer a validated personality assessment, such as the Hogan Personality Inventory, to assess the prospect's personality and leadership style and how she would support effective team interaction.

6. When speaking to references, ask specific questions about team behavior. Ask references to describe how the prospect gets along with fellow team members. Ask for examples of how the prospect argues or debates issues during team sessions. A good idea is to ask the extent to which the prospect plays politics among fellow team members.

Understand Team Processes

Tuckman's (1965) well-known concept of forming, storming, norming, and performing is an easy-to-remember phrase describing how teams form and function. A more current view suggests that teams actually process their activities through two major steps—transition and action. Exhibit 13.1 shows these two activities and how they drive a team toward its goals. The two steps are tied to team goals. Knowing how these major functions work and the challenges they bring can be the key to achieving team success. Morgeson, DeRue, and Karam (2010, 7) write, "As teams work across the transition and action phases they encounter numerous challenges that arise from the

Exhibit 13.1 How Teams Accomplish Their Goals

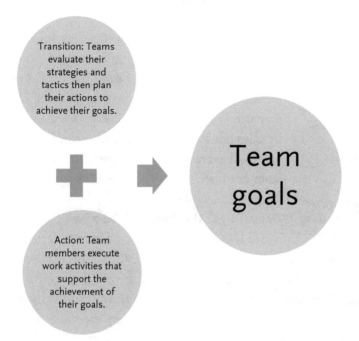

team, organization, and environmental contexts in which the team is operating. These challenges can threaten team viability and make it difficult for them to accomplish their goals, in part because the challenges make it difficult for teams to regulate their goal-directed behavior." The next several suggestions help prevent these problems.

Discuss Team's Value and Values

All team members should learn their individual roles and expectations, evaluate their personal worth to the team, and participate in establishing the values that drive team interactions and behaviors. Doing so improves relationships and cooperation. Because team members are often so busy with their own daily activities, they may fail to invest the necessary time to fully grow and develop as a unit. The team atmosphere should encourage spirited but respectful debate, because better decisions emerge through this exchange.

Under an autocratic CEO, open discussion is unlikely to occur. Teams under such a leader are formed merely to fulfill an organizational convention. Members cannot, nor do they know how to, partake in actual decision making. As a result, members are not aware of their roles and importance. Of course, the underlying problem in this scenario is the leader; however, such a team can be salvaged by a new leader, who can ingrain the values of teamwork with constant dialogue and team exercises.

Demonstrate the Value of "Teaming"

Team leaders must involve all members in setting achievable short-term goals. Achievement of these goals demonstrates the team's value and contribution to improving the organization. An effective leader can demonstrate the value of teaming by bringing tough issues to the group and asking every member to suggest solutions and alternatives. Too often, leaders prefer to handle especially difficult problems themselves or to delegate them to a small subset of the senior management team. Exhibit 13.2 lists strategies for increasing team member participation.

Determine the Purpose of the Team

Unfortunately, many teams do not know why they exist. When asked, most teams respond with, "We share information" or "We discuss strategy," while some say (perhaps mistakenly), "We run the organization."

Ideally, the team, as a unit, should determine its purpose; however, the leader could establish it as well. This purpose provides a framework for what the team must accomplish, so it must be clear and must be understood by every team member. Clarity of purpose prevents the team from taking on activities and goals (or prospective members) that are vague or inappropriate.

Exhibit 13.2 How to Increase Team Member Participation

Establish a clear connection between the team's purpose and activities and the organization's mission and vision. Members need to know not only what they are doing but also how their individual tasks tie in with the bigger goals.

Forge personal relationships with members. Genuine camaraderie is built on members' familiarity with each other's personal interests and pursuits.

Allow and encourage informal discussions (e.g., dialogue about children, movies, personal interests) before or after team meetings. Occasionally, food may be brought in or the group could conduct the meeting over an off-site lunch.

Reward and recognize hard work and accomplishments. A portion of the organization's incentive program should be allotted for team bonuses. If this policy is not an option, the team leader should plan and provide some other form of celebration.

Make team decisions within the confines of team meetings. Members must be present during deliberations and when a final decision is made; merely announcing the decision to the team will harm team morale and discourage future involvement of its members.

Treat all members equally. No one member should be a favorite, regardless of how frequently that person volunteers and how much that person contributes to the team function.

Engage in Team-Building Exercises

Any exercise that confirms the collective strength of the team, assesses the dynamics of the team, and aids in the interaction among members is beneficial. Common team exercises range from simple personality assessment tools (e.g., Myers-Briggs Type Indicator, DiSc) to more sophisticated assessments (e.g., Hogan Personality Inventory; Hogan Development Survey; Hogan Motives, Values, Preferences Inventory) to extensive physical activities (e.g., Outward Bound).

Several years ago, I led a senior management team retreat. Before the retreat, I met individually with team members to ask them the following questions:

- What are the primary reasons for the existence of this senior management team?
- What are the primary reasons for the meetings of this senior management team?
- Does the content of the meetings support the primary reason for the existence of the team?

The responses were varied, but most members indicated that their reason for being was to "collectively lead the organization."

During the retreat, it was revealed that team meetings were show-and-tell sessions, not the mutual interaction that members envisioned. This revelation led to an in-depth discussion about the need to (1) shape and follow a clear purpose and (2) restructure meeting patterns. The team decided to meet every other week solely to discuss strategy and to meet weekly to discuss day-to-day operations.

This team, save for a few members who left to pursue other opportunities, remains intact today. The members report being closer and managing conflicts more effectively.

These exercises offer practical knowledge and skills in a fun and relaxed environment. A note of caution is in order: The person who plans these activities must be an expert on the group's methods, team-building techniques, and objectives. Having a neutral third party to lead the team through these exercises is usually preferable—otherwise, the program could become an expensive time waster for all involved, or worse, could cause irreparable harm in team dynamics.

Confront Relationship and Conduct Issues

Conflicts between team members should be expected. Sometimes such clashes require the leader to intervene, such as when they create disruptions in team functioning. Other times, however, the team itself will police behaviors, discuss ways to stem the conflict, and dole out appropriate punishment if necessary.

Developing a team code of conduct is a valuable team-building exercise. Not only is this activity cooperative, but it also delineates the rules that protect members and monitor their behavior and interactions. Many senior management teams work together on a team code of conduct during their retreats. Exhibit 13.3 is an example of team conduct expectations; this code has been adopted by many healthcare organizations and is currently used by a midwestern health system. Another example, albeit focused on physician practices and developed by the American Medical Association, can be found at www. stepsforward.org/modules/conducting-effective-team-meetings.

Match Words with Actions

A team leader's words and actions carry greater weight than those of members. As such, the leader has to ensure that her behaviors are consistent with her messages, and both must be consistent with the organization's mission, vision, and values. Any discrepancies team members observe could, at best, become fodder for gossip and,

---

Exhibit 13.3 Example of a Senior Management Team Code of Conduct

- Each of us has a right to his own opinion and has the right to state it. Each of us expects that others will carefully and respectfully listen to our opinion and seriously consider it before rejecting it.

- Although our CEO has the authority to make unilateral decisions, she will engage all of us in giving input in as many issues as possible. We respect her right to "some days count the votes and some days weigh the votes."

- We recognize that some decisions are better made with subsets of our team. However, except in unusual situations, we agree that these decisions will not be finalized until the entire team is notified and has the chance to provide final input.

- Each of us has the right to campaign for our issues outside of team meetings and meet individually with other team members to petition for support. However, we agree to tell the team that this campaigning has been done.

- Mystery, intrigue, and politics are fatal diseases. We will strive for openness, honesty, and tact.

The organizational
team-based structure
is an important way for
organizations to remain
competitive by responding
quickly and adapting to
constant, rapid changes.

—Peter G. Northouse
(2016)

at worst, weaken the trust and respect the leader worked hard to establish. It could decimate the participative way of the team, with members perceiving that the leader only preaches about cooperation and sharing but does not really practice these team concepts.

Even in informal interactions, the leader must be watchful of his body language and casual banter to ensure that he remains appropriate, professional, and a role model for others on his team.

A classic example of how *not* to be a leader is Nathan Jessup, the fictitious well-decorated lieutenant colonel played by actor Jack Nicholson in the 1992 movie *A Few Good Men.* Here is how Colonel Jessup defends his leadership: "I have neither the time nor the inclination to explain myself to a man who rises and sleeps under the blanket of the very freedom I provide, then questions the manner in which I provide it! I'd rather you just said thank you and went on your way." Although Colonel Jessup has achieved much, he is not someone a team will choose as, or be proud to call, its leader.

Challenge the Current Boundaries

The hierarchy in every organization creates boundaries, including the following (Band 1994):

- Boundaries of authority—who is in charge of what?
- Boundaries of task—who does what?
- Boundaries of politics—what is our payoff?
- Boundaries of identity—who are we as a group?

Although boundaries are necessary, they can impede decision making and workflow. The leader must allow team members to challenge these boundaries when necessary by setting "must" (critical) and "should" (recommended) guidelines. For example, the team *must* first gain approval from department directors before implementing a process, but the team *should* include all levels of employees in decision making. In this way, the team knows which boundaries are off-limits and which are flexible. To promote cooperation, one leader tells his team: "I expect all of you to work together as though you had authority over the entire organization. Leave your claims of functional turf at the door."

This balance is often difficult. Hughes, Ginnett, and Curphy (2015, 502–3) describe organizations with a hierarchical culture as ones that have "formalized rules and procedures; they tend to be highly structured places to work. Following standard operating procedures, or SOPs, is the rule of the day. The emphasis is on ensuring continuing efficiency, smooth functioning, and dependable operations."

CONCLUSION

Decision making, problem-solving, brainstorming, planning, and implementation are activities that are most effective when executed by a team, not by one person alone. Cooperation and sharing are team traits that do not happen without an open dialogue among team members and without support from the team leader.

Self-Evaluation Questions

❏ Has my team ever discussed its purpose?

❏ Do my team members truly believe in the value of teams?

❏ Do they believe in the value of team deliberations?

❏ Does my team regularly participate in team-building activities?

Cases

Case 13.1

Malcolm Holcomb is the new CEO at a medical center. The agenda for his first meeting with the senior management team includes the following questions:

- What has been the primary purpose of the senior management meetings in the past? What was discussed? What was accomplished?

- What do you want to be the primary purpose of these meetings moving forward? What should we discuss? What should we accomplish?

- What meeting format do you prefer? Do you think that format will enable us to better meet our goals?

- Do each of you have a clear understanding of your roles? Do each of you help one another? How much cooperation and sharing should we expect from this team?

Case 13.1 Questions

1. You are one of Malcolm's vice presidents. How would you answer these questions?

2. Should Malcolm discuss these questions privately with each senior management member *before* raising them in the full group meeting (and therefore getting more open feedback than in an open meeting)? If so, how should he proceed after these private meetings?

Case 13.2

Cynthia Jonas is the CEO of a large suburban community hospital. Her senior leadership team is made up of 17 people, 5 of whom report directly to Cynthia; the rest report to the chief operations officer. Every Tuesday, the entire 17-member team meets for two hours, and often the meetings run longer by about another hour.

During the meeting, Cynthia gives a summary of all the meetings she attended in the previous week. Then, she turns to the chief medical officer (CMO) to discuss physician issues and to the chief financial officer (CFO) to discuss the budget. During these conversations, no one else but Cynthia poses questions and comments to the CMO and the CFO. The rest of the group stays silent or prepares their own reports.

By the time Cynthia ends her conversation with the CMO and CFO, only 15 to 30 minutes are left. The team members then go around the table to give their respective department or project updates. Most team members use this time to tout their accomplishments, but no one pauses for congratulations or recognitions, as time is running out. During these updates, Cynthia is on her laptop, checking e-mail or answering correspondence. Occasionally, she asks for clarification or offers advice.

Recently, Cynthia hired Luann Crosby, an executive coach. Luann sat through one of these meetings. Afterward, Luann pulled Cynthia aside.

LUANN. You know there was a problem with that meeting, right?

CYNTHIA. What do you mean? They're a little long, but no one complains about them.

Case 13.2 Questions
1. You are Luann. Give Cynthia an extensive diagnosis of the meeting. Include as many details in your diagnosis as possible.

(continued)

(continued from previous page)

2. Give Cynthia specific recommendations on improving the meeting.

3. How will you get Cynthia to buy into your suggestion? How will you coach her to gain buy-in from her team?

REFERENCES

Band, W. A. 1994. "Touchstones: Ten New Ideas Revolutionizing Business." In *Organizational Behavior*, 4th ed., edited by R. Kreiter and A. Kinicki. New York: Richard D. Irwin.

Hughes, R. L., R. C. Ginnett, and G. J. Curphy. 2015. *Leadership: Enhancing the Lessons of Experience*, 8th ed. Burr Ridge, IL: McGraw-Hill Education.

Katzenbach, J. R., and D. K. Smith. 1993. *The Wisdom of Teams: Creating the High-Performance Organization*. Boston: Harvard Business School Press.

Morgeson, F. P., D. S. DeRue, and E. P. Karam. 2010. "Leadership in Teams: A Functional Approach to Understanding Leadership Structures and Processes." *Journal of Management* 36 (1): 5–39.

Northouse, P. G. 2016. *Leadership: Theory and Practice*, 7th ed. Los Angeles: SAGE Publications.

Tuckman, B. W. 1965. "Developmental Sequence in Small Groups." *Psychological Bulletin* 63 (6): 384–99.

SUGGESTED READINGS

Collins, C. G., C. B. Gibson, N. R. Quigley, and S. K. Parker. 2016. "Unpacking Team Dynamics with Growth Modeling: An Approach to Test, Refine, and Integrate Theory." *Organizational Psychology Review* 6 (1): 63–91.

De Cooman, R., T. Vantilborgh, M. Bal, and X. Lub. 2016. "Creating Inclusive Teams Through Perceptions of Supplementary and Complementary Person–Team Fit: Examining the Relationship Between Person–Team Fit and Team Effectiveness." *Group Organization Management* 41 (3): 310–42.

Lanaj, K., and J. R. Hollenbeck. 2015. "Leadership Over-emergence in Self-managing Teams: The Role of Gender and Countervailing Biases." *Academy of Management Journal* 58 (5): 1476–94.

Owens, B. P., and D. R. Hekman. 2016. "How Does Leader Humility Influence Team Performance? Exploring the Mechanisms of Contagion and Collective Promotion Focus." *Academy of Management Journal* 59 (3): 1088–11.

Weer, C. H., M. S. DiRenzo, and F. M. Shipper. 2016. "A Holistic View of Employee Coaching: Longitudinal Investigation of the Impact of Facilitative and Pressure-Based Coaching on Team Effectiveness." *Journal of Applied Behavioral Science* 52 (2): 187–214.

CHAPTER 14

Cohesiveness and Collaboration

Team-based organizations have faster response capability because of their flatter organizational structures, which rely on teams and new technology to enable communication across time and space.

—Peter G. Northouse (2016)

AT A FOCUS group during a leadership conference, Rakesh Jaya, facilitator and organizational development researcher, asked participants from different organizations to explain the structure and results of their own senior management meetings.

JAMES SMITH, CHIEF OPERATIONS OFFICER. All of our meetings are preplanned and highly structured. We don't meet unless there's a clear reason for it. We follow the agenda strictly and honor the time allotment for each agenda item. A detailed follow-up list is prepared at the conclusion of every meeting. Everyone is required to come well prepared for his or her reports and to participate in all the discussions.

MELANIE RODRIGUEZ, CHIEF EXECUTIVE OFFICER. Our team meets every two weeks, and the meetings last for four to six hours. Long ago, the team collectively decided that we wouldn't use an agenda because it's too limiting. Our meetings are open-ended, so we have the freedom to explore and deliberate on an issue fully. We arrive at many of our decisions this way, and we think this is a creative approach to thinking about and resolving our problems. We realize that this structure is not for everyone, so only the senior-level members of our team are invited to the meetings. But we do provide a summary of our discussions to the rest of the team, and they are encouraged to speak to their vice presidents if they have any concerns or comments.

AMY BRODERICK, CHIEF FINANCIAL OFFICER. I work for a large system, and our team is composed of 25 members. Every week, the chief executives from our nine hospitals meet for two hours to discuss strategic issues. Each of these meetings is focused on one issue and is led by a sponsor. This way, all team members have an opportunity to run a meeting and be well informed about at least one strategy. Then, every month, the entire 25-person team meets to exchange reports about business unit outcomes, ongoing and upcoming strategic initiatives, and some operations-related issues. If needed, we invite staff outside of the team to provide input and share information.

STEVE MICHAEL, SENIOR VICE PRESIDENT OF COMMUNICATIONS AND MARKETING. We built subgroups into our team to increase our efficiency and effectiveness. The subgroups meet every week, and they report their discussions and decisions to the full team when we all meet twice each month. Our CEO trusts our judgment and skills, so she gives us much autonomy but expects us to be accountable for our outcomes. Before the start of our monthly meeting, we open with a breakfast and the CEO says with a huge smile on her

> face, "Tell me something I don't know," then people start talking about their children's wedding or a movie they just saw. There's always an opportunity for us to get to know each other in a more personal way. We all know and respect each other, and I think that because of that we offer help to those who are struggling with their operations or projects.

MANY LEADERSHIP TEAMS in healthcare strive to capture the entrepreneurial spirit of successful businesses. This spirit makes a team cohesive, as it cheers team members on through conception, development, rollout, and marketing of new products or services. Unfortunately, this spirit is temporary and can be undermined by old-fashioned jealousy and selfish tendencies.

When a business expands its operation, new members are added to the existing team. Although a logical move, this addition could be destructive to the cohesiveness of the team, as current and new members feel tension or quarrel over whose ideas are better, who has the power to make decisions, who is responsible for which tasks, or what improvements need to be pursued (or not pursued). As the rift grows, member support for the common goal diminishes. Although cohesiveness increases team productivity, morale, and camaraderie, it does not prevent schism brought on by territorial battles and other issues. Exhibit 14.1 lists the downsides to cohesiveness.

Collaboration, on the other hand, pulls together divided parties to work toward a mutually accepted goal. It transcends traditional compromise in that no exchange of services is necessary to achieve the preferred outcomes of both parties; it demands only equal input and dedication to the cause. Most important, collaboration often results in conflict resolution.

> Team members (in shared leadership) step forward when situations warrant, providing the leadership necessary, and then step back to allow others to lead. Such shared leadership has become more and more important in today's organizations to allow faster responses to more complex issues.
>
> —Peter G. Northouse (2016)

Exhibit 14.1 Disadvantages of Team Cohesiveness

Low performance norms and poor performers. Performance norms are the standards expected from all team members. They dictate the quality and quantity of work—how vigorous, effective, and productive the work is; what goals should be achieved; and what contributions should be tendered. In a cohesive environment, these norms (primarily unwritten) are low. Highly competent members pick up the slack (perhaps even gladly) for members who have subpar abilities. As a result, those who need skills improvement remain undeveloped and dependent on the high achievers. In a contentious environment, however, low performance norms become a source of conflict. The best performers resent the fact that they have to cover for the poor performers. Worse, many competent members are too polite to deliver constructive criticism.

Proliferation of groupthink. Groupthink is, simply, unanimous thinking. When the team is cohesive, its members tend to lose their individual perspectives. As a result, new and creative thoughts are blocked off, objections are stifled, and concurrence becomes the standard. Instead of pursuing the goals of the organization as a whole, keeping the solidarity of the team becomes the team's main purpose.

Low tolerance for change. Founding team members are loyal to the initial team purpose, composition, rules, norms, and goals they helped establish. They believe that these components strengthen team cohesiveness, which is given high value. As such, they are uncomfortable with change, even when they recognize that evolution could improve team functions. New members are often viewed as disruptive outsiders and detrimental to the cohesiveness of the team.

Team goals take precedence over organizational goals. A highly cohesive team is fanatical about the welfare of its members. Some leadership teams have reduced clinical and support staff but maintained administrators. Some have paid executive bonuses despite financially tight years, a practice that has gained significant public disapproval.

Conflicting parties typically respond in one of the following ways:

- Avoid the other party and thus the conflict
- Give in to the demands of the other party

- Compete, with the goal to win
- Compromise or strike a deal
- Collaborate, with a goal to achieve

Consider the last three approaches. Competition is never an appropriate response because it amplifies the damage and makes it irreversible. Historically, compromise was often recommended, but it leaves both parties only partially satisfied and distorts the quid pro quo practice of "saving" favors (see chapter 15) to be redeemed in a later conflict. If neither party anticipates future dealings with one another, then a compromise is usually a better approach than collaboration. Conversely, if the parties continue their relationship and expect further dispute, then collaboration is the only responsible solution. The latter situation is the case with senior leadership teams.

Cohesiveness begets collaboration, and collaboration begets cohesiveness. Although one can exist without the other, one cannot be as effective without the other.

THE CONCEPT IN PRACTICE

Despite its disadvantages, cohesiveness is an important component of collaboration. The following methods can help in forming a cohesive and collaborative team.

Minimize Selfish Behavior

In teams, selfishness is a contagious disease that can easily spread to all members. The team leader, as the role model, must demonstrate that she works on behalf of others' interests, not just her own. If not, team members will suspect the leader's motives and cohesiveness will decline. The leader is also responsible for confronting members who contribute only to advance their own pursuits, not the team's. Appropriate team behavior must be established and put in writing—possibly during a retreat (see discussion about team code of conduct in chapter 13).

Assess the Size of the Team

Mergers and acquisitions, new service lines, and corporate partnerships extend the reach of an organization's leadership team and expand its size. As new members and responsibilities are added, the team loses its camaraderie and cohesiveness. A team that has more than 11 or 12 members often experiences a split, whereby the members form their own factions because they cannot find a commonality among the entire group. In a large team, the members also do not receive enough individual attention.

The generally accepted principle is that the team should have between 6 and 11 members. However, there is no ideal size. Here are several important considerations for setting the team size:

- If the task is repetitive, the team may have many members.
- If the task is complex, a large team can slow down the decision-making process.
- If a lot of collaboration is required, teams larger than 11 or 12 members can create problems.

If reducing the team size is not an option, the leader could manage perception about the size through the following approaches:

- Divide operations executives and strategy executives into two teams.
- Hold less frequent meetings with the entire team, but convene subgroups more often.
- Do not replace a team member when turnover occurs.

Get to Know One Another

Team leaders should socialize with members at every opportunity presented, including before or after meetings, organizational events, and informal celebrations. These interactions not only create a personal bond between the leader and members but also communicate that the leader is interested in the person behind the executive.

Consider the following bonding practices by several successful leaders:

- Every fourth Friday, one CEO takes her senior management team to an off-site location for a full-day retreat. The first half (from breakfast until lunch) of the retreat is dedicated to business and operations. The second half is reserved for non-work-related matters, such as getting-to-know-you exercises.
- After its monthly meeting with the board, one leadership team spends the day at an off-site location to enjoy each other's company and catch up. The different venue serves to refocus the team and inspire creativity.
- One CEO holds a weekly no-agenda lunch session with his team, allowing team members to interact with one another in an informal setting.

Minimize the Influence of Cliques

Unfortunately, cliques are not confined to junior high school; they are prevalent in the workplace as well. The larger the organization, the larger the teams; the larger the team, the greater the possibility of cliques forming. Cliques are detrimental to any team because they represent cohesiveness without collaboration. That is, such groups are powerful because of their solidarity and focus on a common goal, but members of cliques fail or even refuse to partner with others to achieve that objective. Thus, they alienate others and disrupt the normal function of a team.

The leader can address the challenges of cliques in the team in several ways:

1. *Occasionally acknowledge the clique's existence during team meetings.* For example, one CEO announces (only half-jokingly), "I already know that the operations people have come to a conclusion on this matter a long time ago. Now I want to know what they talked about before this meeting!" By publicly recognizing the clique, the leader is making it clear that side negotiations will not be tolerated.

2. *Confront the clique privately.* Generally, a clique engenders negativity among team members because it has its own agenda. Divide and conquer could be one of the approaches a clique can use to sway the opinion of team members who are undecided about a certain decision or plan. By confronting the clique, the leader is directly appealing to its sense of propriety while strongly emphasizing the need to work together, not sabotage, team efforts. This confrontation must be done calmly so as not to widen the rift between the team and the clique.

3. *Assign clique members to a task force related to their area of expertise.* The goal of this strategy is to capitalize on the clique's strengths to benefit the team. Many members of

a clique are experts in their fields, and they withhold this knowledge from the team to further their own agendas. If the leader delegates them to a task force specific to their areas—for example, a clinical quality-improvement task force—clique members are more likely to apply their skills and abilities and teach other team members.

4. *Have an open discussion with the entire team about the damage a clique, or any subgroup, can inflict on cohesiveness and collaboration.* Such a discussion (which is a good topic for a retreat) is sensitive and should be done with an expert facilitator.

Discuss and Evaluate the Team's Purpose

Over time, the team's composition changes. As old members leave and new members take their place, the team's reason for being evolves as well. The team must regularly (annually, perhaps) redefine its purpose, reassess its goals, and reestablish its expectations. This discussion must involve all team members, because nothing inspires commitment more than 100 percent participation from those who embody the principles and implement the changes.

Treat All Members Fairly and Equally

An imbalance of power produces divisiveness, which is counter to the ideas of cohesiveness and collaboration. The fact that some members fill higher positions or have more organizational and community clout than do the rest of the team should not affect the way the leader regards all team members.

For example, if two members (say, the chief operations officer and the chief nursing officer)

> Group cohesion is the glue that keeps a group together. It is the sum of the forces that attract members to a group, provide resistance to leaving it, and motivate them to be active in it.
>
> —Richard L. Hughes, Robert C. Ginnett, and Gordon J. Curphy (2015)

commit the same indecent behavior (say, sexual harassment), the leader cannot excuse one but censure the other. Not only will this action spark a protest among the team, but it will also run counter to the service mission of both the team and the organization. The same can be said for personal relationships. The leader cannot pick and choose which member he will befriend or get to know better. Doing so will send a message that the leader plays favorites and will cause team members to distance themselves.

Designate a Team Role for Each Member

A team role is a specific character or function that each member consciously or unconsciously inhabits at any team gathering (e.g., meeting, retreat). Roles include cheerleader, devil's advocate, team conscience, team historian, and meeting planner. A member's personality or professional background lends itself to role assignment. For example, a member who has worked for the organization for 30 years could be named the historian.

Although seemingly simple, the practice of role designation reinforces members' sense of belonging to the group and clarifies their contributions.

Reassess the Compensation Policy

The organization's compensation structure indirectly affects team cohesiveness. That is, if the pay policy is designed primarily to recognize and reward individual performance, the message is that team participation and outcomes are not as valued. As a result, team members may reserve their best work for their own individual projects (the accomplishment of which will yield a bonus or raise) or develop hidden agendas that could conflict with the team's. Although compensation is beyond the purview of this book, money is an important consideration for the leader.

Rally the Team

As detailed in chapter 1, today's executives are faced with multidimensional and interrelated challenges. The most difficult times are always the most opportune times for the leader to pull the team together, especially if the team has experienced infighting and division.

Rallying the team should go beyond vocal cheerleading to boost morale, however. It should be backed up by practices that ease conflict and promote unity. For example, at the end of every meeting, the leader exclaims, "We're a great team! Let's get those quality numbers up!" However, at the next meeting, the leader publicly berates one group for the poor outcomes it achieved while exalting another group for its remarkable performance. Worse, he does not offer guidance or advice to those who are struggling. This leader's mixed message facilitates unhealthy competition, retards collaboration, and discourages improvement. At the end of the day, team members will hear, "We're a great team!," but not believe it.

CONCLUSION

Without cohesiveness and collaboration, a team is merely a collection of people who sit around a conference table when they are told to do so. Such a team produces nothing without difficulty and waste, which in turn cascade to the rest of the organization. More important, this kind of team does not advance the mission and vision of the organization or meet the needs of the community it supposedly serves.

Self-Evaluation Questions

❏ Why does my team meet? What do we accomplish when we meet?

❏ Would outside observers describe my team as cohesive?

❏ Has my team studied collaboration? Have we had training in conflict resolution?

❏ Consider the symptoms of groupthink listed earlier in this chapter. What symptoms does my team exhibit?

Case and Exercise

Case 14.1

St. Nicholas Health System is an integrated health delivery organization comprising St. Nicholas Medical Center, Suburban Western Health Center, Suburban East Health Center, St. Nicholas Employed Physician Practice, St. Nicholas HMO, and St. Nicholas Home Care and Durable Medical Equipment Corporation. The health system operates in a highly competitive city of 2.5 million residents.

Headed by CEO Serena Parris, the leadership group has 25 members, including the executive vice president and chief operations officer (EVP/COO), several system senior vice presidents, assorted system vice presidents, and the site administrators from each business unit. The senior team meets weekly to discuss tactical and strategic operations as well as ongoing projects (if time allows, which is rare).

The site administrators do not feel they are part of the executive team, given that they report to the COO and not to the CEO, and that most of the discussions relate to the system rather than the individual business units. In fact, at St. Nicholas, much of the work is accomplished through interactions between the vice presidents or executive directors and administrators or middle managers. Because Serena is a hands-off leader, she has given her EVP/COO freedom to make ongoing operations decisions. The EVP/COO gives the site administrators much autonomy to run their own facilities.

Serena depends heavily on only three executives on the team—the EVP/COO, the senior vice president of medical affairs, and the chief financial officer. The rest of the 25-member team is aware that Serena has frequent daily communications with these three executives.

Case 14.1 Questions

1. What are the strengths of this team? Its weaknesses?

2. Do the site administrators belong to this group? Explain your answer.

3. What message does Serena send to her team by relying so much on three team members over everyone else?

4. If you were a consultant, what advice would you offer Serena to strengthen the team?

Exercise 14.1

Some leadership experts argue that members of the senior management team independently work on their own issues and come together only occasionally to coordinate organizational activities and set organizational strategy.

Consider the following thoughts regarding the work of senior leaders and their teams:

(continued)

(continued from previous page)

1. The job of a typical healthcare vice president has an individual focus. That is, she spends most of her time on activities that have nothing to do with the work of the senior management team of which she is a member.

2. Working challenges faced at the middle management and frontline supervisory levels are usually short-term in nature (there is an immediacy to the nature of the issue), and the problems that must be solved are usually clearer. Issues at the senior management level are much grayer, involving strategy and longer-term decisions.

3. Compared with the problems faced by middle management, the challenges encountered by the senior management team require strategic (not operational), long-term responses. Similarly, the purpose of a senior management team (e.g., achieve a 4 percent margin) is more abstract than the purpose of any other organizational team.

4. Senior-level leaders have two, often overlapping, performance goals—a corporate goal and an individual goal.

5. At the senior leadership level, complementary skills are less important than position. In true team situations, the extra performance capability that a real team provides comes mostly from its complementary skills—that is, executives with clinical backgrounds are knowledgeable about patient care operations, while leaders with financial backgrounds are adept at business concepts.

6. Establishing and maintaining team standards of behavior are difficult for a senior management team because this group meets less frequently than do other teams.

7. Members of senior management teams are not "mutually accountable" to each other; rather, they are individually accountable to the CEO. Mutual accountability is hard to establish because one executive has too many responsibilities.

Exercise 14.1 Questions
1. If these points are correct, how should senior executives enhance their working effectiveness? Can executives create real teams?

2. If you were starting an organization from scratch, how would you assemble the leadership team?

REFERENCES

Hughes, R. L., R. C. Ginnett, and G. J. Curphy. 2015. *Leadership: Enhancing the Lessons of Experience*, 8th ed. Burr Ridge, IL: McGraw-Hill Education.

Northouse, P. G. 2016. *Leadership: Theory and Practice*, 7th ed. Los Angeles: SAGE Publications.

SUGGESTED READINGS

Cohn, K. H. 2008. "Collaborative Co-mentoring." Healthcare Collaboration. Published June 18. www.healthcarecollaboration.com/collaborative-co-mentoring/.

Homberg, F., and H. T. M. Bui. 2013. "Top Management Team Diversity: A Systematic Review." *Group and Organization Management* 38 (4): 455–79.

Hurt, K. J., and M. A. Abebe. 2015. "The Effect of Conflict Type and Organizational Crisis on Perceived Strategic Decision Effectiveness: An Empirical Investigation." *Journal of Leadership and Organizational Studies* 22 (3): 340–54.

Shaeffner, M., H. Huettermann, D. Gebert, S. Boerner, E. Kearney, and L. J. Song. 2015. "Swim or Sink Together: The Potential of Collective Team Identification and Team Member Alignment for Separating Task and Relationship Conflicts." *Group and Organization Management* 40 (4): 467–99.

Susskind, A. M., and P. R. Odom-Reed. 2016. "Team Members' Centrality, Cohesion, Conflict, and Performance in Multi-University Geographically Distributed Project Teams." *Communication Research*. Published February 3. http://crx.sagepub.com/content/early/2016/01/28/00936502156269 72.abstract.

Weingart, L. R., K. J. Behfar, C. Bendersky, G. Todorova, and K. A. Jehn. 2015. "The Directness and Oppositional Intensity of Conflict Expression." *Academy of Management Review* 40 (2): 235–62.

CHAPTER 15

Trust

When you are not present, people can tell.
When you are, people respond.

—Amy Cuddy (2015)

MAJOR **M**ICHELLE **H**ARRIS, an Army Medical Service Corps
officer, has just returned to the United States from a
third deployment overseas. As a healthcare executive, she is
active in her professional association's local chapter. In one
meeting, she and Chuck Hall, a fellow executive, discuss the
concept of trust in leadership.

CHUCK. Michelle, in your position, it must be great to simply
give orders that your team won't question or distrust. I'd
love to do the same in my hospital. But I have to sell every
idea, earn my colleagues' trust every step of the way.

MICHELLE. No, that's not how it works in the military.[1] There's
a book called *Leadership Lessons from West Point*. It points
out that in the military, trust is even more critical than in
civilian situations.

CHUCK. How so?

MICHELLE. In the military, we ask—note that I say "ask," not "command"—people to put their lives on the line, so we work harder to earn their trust. We provide constant training to ensure high levels of competency and safety. We demonstrate that we care about our personnel, and a high degree of openness can be observed in our training. We have to be on the same page, especially in combat situations. Everyone has a deep understanding of our missions and the dangers and payoffs they present. Movies about the military don't accurately depict the high levels of trust that underlie everything we do.

CHUCK. That's quite impressive. I'd like to invite you to speak to my senior management team next month, if you have time to spare.

TRUST IS THE first value all team members must learn. Without trust, team members engage in fierce competition, backstabbing, and hypocrisy (see exhibit 15.1).

Merriam-Webster's Collegiate Dictionary, Eleventh Edition, defines trust as the "assured reliance on the character, ability, strength, or truth of someone or something." In leadership teams, trust is the members' confidence in each other's ability and resolve to uphold the team's principles and to work toward its goals. It is what allows one member to vote for another's untested, seemingly outlandish proposal. It is what makes members stand behind their leader in moments of failure or scrutiny. Exhibit 15.2 enumerates the essential bases of trust, and exhibit 15.3 is a behavior guideline for all team members to promote a culture of trust.

Cuddy, Kohut, and Neffinger (2013) state that "trust also facilitates the exchange and acceptance of ideas—it allows people to hear others' message—and boosts the quantity and quality of the ideas

Exhibit 15.1 Consequences of Lack of Trust

- Team members keep important and relevant information to themselves for fear that others will steal or sabotage their ideas.
- The team leader or high-ranking team members undermine the suggestions or plans submitted by lower-level members.
- Competition for resources among team members is excessive.
- Side deals or negotiations constantly occur.
- Many team members are deliberately left out of the planning and decision-making processes.
- Cliques have more influence on and power over team members than does the leader.
- Political maneuvering is rampant and viewed as a necessary practice.

Exhibit 15.2 The Five Components of Trust

1. *Integrity*—honesty and truthfulness

2. *Competence*—technical and interpersonal knowledge and skills

3. *Consistency*—reliability, predictability, and good judgment

4. *Loyalty*—willingness to support, protect, and save someone else

5. *Openness*—willingness to share ideas and information freely

Source: Adapted from Robbins and Judge (2013).

that are produced within an organization. Most important, trust provides the opportunity to change people's attitudes and beliefs, not just their outward behavior."

An exchange of tangible or intangible favors or goodwill is common practice among team members. This transaction is modeled after the economics of bartering or the *social exchange theory*. This theory posits that individuals decide the fairness of a relationship on the basis of a self-measured give–take ratio. If a person thinks he

Exhibit 15.3 How Team Members Can Engender Trust

Speak your mind. The truth could hurt, but it could also pave a path for improved and increased communication. Be calm while you express yourself, and be receptive to the responses.

Maintain confidentiality. A lot of leadership team matters are confidential, and for good reason. Such matters, including informal or casual conversations, must not be discussed or shared.

Actively support the team. Do not refer to or speak about the team negatively, inside or outside the team setting. People's poor perception of the team extends to their poor perception of you, if only because you belong to the group.

Embrace openness. Trust develops in an open and candid environment.

Practice due process. In the team setting, due process means that all team members have the right to be heard fairly.

---

is giving more than he is receiving, he will perceive the exchange as unfair, and thus he may withdraw from giving. Conversely, if the person believes the things he gives and receives are of comparable value, he will continue the exchange relationship. The same idea is true of trust: It is a commodity that team members can exchange.

Unlike other favors, however, trust is not easily earned. A team member must prove her trustworthiness to the rest of the group by showing and having faith and concern; being transparent and accountable; providing support, assistance, information, and resources; and aligning with the general consensus without sacrificing personal values. More important, the team member must display these behaviors consistently and over time.

Once earned, trust must be maintained.

When team members cease to trade trust, a "depression" occurs, prohibiting members from cooperating, sharing information, and collaborating. It harms the cohesiveness of the unit and ultimately leads to various dysfunctions.

THE CONCEPT IN PRACTICE

The following approaches can enhance trustworthiness and trust levels among team members.

Acknowledge the Quid Pro Quo Practice

Honesty engenders trust. By publicly recognizing and discussing the fact that favors are exchanged to help forward the team's initiatives, team members can use that fact to achieve the most optimal outcomes. The concept may be woven into trust-building exercises.

Earn, Do Not Expect, Trust

Trust does not develop overnight, especially in a field such as healthcare that is in a constant state of flux. A leader cannot order her team members to trust her, nor can she think that trust comes automatically with the position. She must first assess her true self and either improve or maintain her trustworthiness. Trust building is a multistep and multiyear journey that can be easily derailed by a small move in the wrong direction.

> People want to feel understood by their leaders. Trust comes before strength and it becomes a conduit of influence. Your strength is a little bit threatening before people trust you. But when they trust you and you are their leader, it's a gift to them. Presence allows you to build that trust because you are saying, "I'm here, I care about you. I'm listening and what I am telling you to do is not just based on my own personal opinion but what I'm observing and hearing from you."
>
> —Amy Cuddy (quoted in Schawbel 2016)

Display Consistent Behavior

In some respects, trust is about predictability and consistency. Team members will be hard-pressed to have confidence in a leader who does not do what he says or is fickle, temperamental, indecisive, impulsive, or too spontaneous. Moreover, followers are discouraged

An understanding of
people and relationships
requires an understanding
of trust. Trust requires
the coexistence of two
converging beliefs.
When I believe you are
competent and that you
care about me, I will trust
you. Competency alone
or caring by itself will not
engender trust. Both are
necessary.

—Peter R. Scholtes (1998)

when the leader's words and deeds are contradictory. For example, one CEO declares that he wants to create a culture of empowerment, but he insists on reviewing everyone's work all the time and giving the final approval on every single decision. An erratic or unpredictable leader is viewed as unreliable and hence not deserving of trust.

Drive Out Fear

In his well-known book, *The Five Dysfunctions of a Team*, Patrick Lencioni (2002, 43) presents a pyramid that shows his theory of the five types of dysfunction. Notably, he puts lack of trust at the bottom of the pyramid, indicating that it is the most serious of the five. Most readers would agree that when trust is absent in the work culture (or any culture for that matter), uncertainty and ultimately fear can easily develop.

Clearly, fear has no place on any team. Following are some strategies for driving fear away:

- Establish and sustain a culture in which people can express opinions, concerns, suggestions, and even dissent without putting their jobs, reputation, undertaking, or team membership in jeopardy.

- Do not discuss or negotiate anything in secret. Confidentiality is markedly different from secrecy, and the latter breeds suspicions, gossip, and disloyalty. Secrets are always revealed, and when they are, team members feel left out and threatened. Everyone on the team must practice transparency.

- Persuade members to participate in team activities. One leader holds "Think Out Loud" meetings, where the team brainstorms ideas. The goal of this session is to stimulate creative thinking and generate novel approaches to old challenges.

- Be accessible. The executive suite should not be a hiding spot; it should be one of the places a leader can be found, in addition to the hallways, patient care units, conference rooms, cafeterias, other people's work spaces, and so on. Presence at organizational events and community functions as well as the availability of contact information are two ways a leader can become more accessible.

Avoid the Perception and Reality of Conflict of Interest

Many situations in healthcare present a conflict-of-interest challenge because healthcare delivery and management entail so many types of exchanges, some of which could work in the self-interest of those involved in the exchange.

Full disclosure is one way to combat the perception of a conflict of interest. For example, the Cleveland Clinic now publicizes the business dealings of its physicians and other clinicians with drug and medical device makers. In April 2009, the Institute of Medicine issued the report *Conflict of Interest in Medical, Research, Education and Practice* (Office of News and Public Information 2009). The report discusses how "disclosure by physicians and researchers not only to their employers but also to other medical organizations of their financial links to pharmaceutical, biotechnology, and medical device firms is an essential first step in identifying and managing conflicts of interest and needs to be improved."

Many healthcare organizations, including professional associations and healthcare businesses, already have a conflict-of-interest policy in place. However, more needs to be done in this area to minimize (if not eliminate) the risk of conflict of interest and its subsequent consequences to the reputation of the organization, its leaders, and its staff.

Be Candid

Candor is the sincerity and frankness of speech and behavior. It runs counter to lying, condescending, or exaggerating. Speaking candidly means

- retaining eye contact and a steady voice,
- stating facts and withholding opinions that could hurt,
- focusing on the situation and not going off on a tangent,
- inviting questions or comments, and
- giving the other person a chance to respond.

Retreats are optimal moments for candid discussions, as John Kotter (1996, 132) proposes in his book *Leading Change*: "Most of the time must be spent encouraging honest discussion about how individuals think and feel with regard to the organization, its problems and opportunities. Communication channels between people are opened or strengthened. Mutual understanding is enlarged. Intellectual and social activities are designed to encourage the growth of trust."

> Trust in a relationship generally develops gradually over time through the course of personal interaction. Taking some kind of risk in relation to the other person and feeling you weren't injured (emotionally or physically) in the process is what moves trust to new levels.
>
> —James M. Kouzes and Barry Z. Posner (2003)

Unfortunately, many team members recoil from voicing their opinions and concerns in front of the whole team, as my experience with leading senior management retreats has shown. Although these members were willing to be candid with me in private, they preferred not to speak when faced by the other members. To combat this phenomenon, I started meeting individually with team members before the retreat. I emphasized the merits of being open and honest, and I recruited them to contribute to the group dialogue. Also, I occasionally brought a list of concerns, with permission from the team, to serve as a starting point for our candid discussion.

Use Finesse

Finesse does not cost anything, but it is worth a small fortune. However, like a battery, finesse is negatively and positively charged. Dealing with someone with decorum and courtesy is a plus, but it can also be a minus: It can prohibit the confrontation needed to reveal underlying conflicts. For example, a cohesive leadership team that has been together for many years and has rarely argued over issues does not take kindly to confrontation. As suggested in chapter 14, a cohesive team does not necessarily make a productive team because many of its members have grown complacent; thus, the team can use a little shake-up once in a while. Having tact, however, prevents boorish behavior.

> High-performance teams are characterized by high mutual trust among members. That is, members believe in the integrity, character, and ability of each other. But as you know from personal relationships, trust is fragile. It takes a long time to build, can be easily destroyed, and is hard to regain. Also, since trust begets trust and distrust begets distrust, maintaining trust requires careful attention by management.
>
> —Stephen P. Robbins and Timothy A. Judge (2013)

Expect and Welcome Resistance

The process of earning trust—essentially, being open—puts a person in a vulnerable position. The leader (or a team member) should be prepared for criticism, doubt, resistance, and reluctance but should not take these responses personally. One CEO puts this risk in perspective: "If you want trust within your management group, you have to expect to get shot down sometimes. Then you get back up, thank the person who shot you, and move on."

Do Not Take Advantage

A leadership position offers many opportunities for inappropriate conduct. Sadly, in the past decade alone, high-level executives in and out of the healthcare field have exploited this truth. Taking advantage for the purpose of personal gain is wrong in any situation, as this act almost always has a victim. A leader could keep herself from taking advantage by obeying the golden rule of bartering: The exchange must be of equal value.

Grant Authority Appropriately

The power to bestow decision-making capabilities on team members falls on the leader, so he must exercise extreme care and judgment. Personal friendships, resentment or anger over past insults, and even lack of information can cloud the leader's ability to grant this authority. A poor choice can lead to infighting, charges of favoritism, and resistance. It could also erode the leader's trustworthiness. The best defense against such a scenario is always awareness and wisdom, which can come from being fully present physically, mentally, and emotionally.

Understand the Links Between Trust and Mission and Action

As this chapter's opening vignette indicates, military operations exemplify how trust is the basis of mission fulfillment. Trust essentially powers the actions that support the mission. Without trust, the action either does not occur or is performed haphazardly, causing grave harm. As retired Major General David Rubenstein, FACHE (2016), states:

> The first thing that comes to mind when talking about trust is the chain of events that occur in the Army from words to actions to trust to mission accomplishment. A soldier will hear his or her leader's words but waits to see the leader's actions. When action matches words, the soldier starts to build a trust that says, "I'll go in harm's way to do my job because I trust you." When I hand my static line to the jumpmaster, 800 feet

above the ground on a moonless night, I'm saying, "I'm ready to jump out of this plane because I trust you've ensured that my equipment and I are ready."

CONCLUSION

Trust is the assurance of goodwill between two people. It builds over time and must not be taken for granted. Trust among team members is a commodity that can be traded, facilitating ongoing relationships and improving the likelihood of collaboration, cooperation, and sharing of information.

Lacking trust is like walking into a room full of complete strangers. You have a problem: You need to finish an important project, but you have no time to do so. Imagine asking these strangers in the room to help you. Imagine handing them the incomplete work. Imagine sharing with them valuable and confidential information about the project. Imagine encouraging them to collaborate and cooperate with each other. Imagine giving them a quick deadline. Imagine doing all of this without feeling paranoid, doubtful, desperate, exasperated, and doomed.

Self-Evaluation Questions

❑ How is trust displayed among my team members? Do we barter trust, and do we understand its function in the team?

❑ Is my leadership style marked by openness and honesty? Do others easily approach me?

❑ To what extent am I known as a good team player?

❑ Is my communication with the team candid and straightforward? To what extent do I encourage this communication style?

Team Evaluation Questions

To what extent do team members

- ❑ believe in each other's abilities and competence?
- ❑ believe in each other's inclinations and intentions?
- ❑ believe in each other's integrity?
- ❑ get along with each other?
- ❑ share the same goals?
- ❑ rely and depend on each other?
- ❑ have confidence in each other's motives and behaviors?

Cases

Case 15.1

New CEO Doug Wright has a problem. His leadership team displays dysfunctional behaviors. Infighting is rampant, and cooperation and sharing of information are nonexistent. At meetings, most team members do not participate in the discussion, resigned to sitting quietly after they give an update on their respective responsibilities. Recently, two chief executives suddenly quit, leaving the other team members gossiping about the reasons.

Doug has spoken to the team (both as a group and individually) at length about the problem. He has touted the values of openness, honesty, and trust. He has encouraged the team members to speak their minds and has informed them of the no-recrimination policy he has just instituted. But still, the team seems removed, content with doing as it is told.

Frustrated, Doug contacts Roxanne Samanski, an organizational development consultant. The first question he asks her is, "Shall I fire all of them and start fresh?"

Case 15.1 Questions

1. If you were Roxanne, how would you respond to Doug? What suggestions would you offer?

2. What is the role that lack of trust plays in this situation?

3. Do you think it's important to find out the history of this team to understand its current dysfunctions?

Case 15.2

Ralph O'Riley is a dynamic CEO of a large for-profit system. He is well known in the community. He is a brilliant businessman, and he is highly rewarded for it, enjoying various perks such as a beautifully appointed office suite, a company car, and a parking spot right outside of the hospital entrance.

He rarely attends employee-related functions, and he only occasionally visits the other facilities in the system, let alone the units on his own campus. He is a mythical figure among employees and intimidates his own leadership team. He shows up to meetings late, relies on his chief executives to "fill him in on the agenda," and does not know all of his staff members' names or positions. He does not participate in operational discussions, but he gives orders that affect operations, something that confounds his team and angers the rank and file.

Once during a retreat, Ralph was overheard by some of his team members boasting about his golf game and his power. "This is a waste of my time," he complained over his cell phone. "It's not PC to say it, but I own these people. They do what I tell them to do. I made a lot of money for this system. Now they should give me a break."

Case 15.2 Questions

Obviously, everything Ralph is seems to run counter with the practices that build and enhance trust.

(continued)

(continued from previous page)

1. What long-term effects does Ralph's behavior have on his team, the employees at large, and the organization as a whole? Are these effects irreversible?

2. Ralph is clearly a financial wizard and has great business instincts. How should he leverage these competencies to create a better culture? To make himself even more powerful by being approachable and trustworthy?

3. What role does power play in Ralph's success?

NOTE

1. This vignette represents the contributions that military officers bring to healthcare leadership and the healthcare field. It highlights the importance of trust in the military and its applicability to civilian leadership. Attendees at American College of Healthcare Executives events (especially the annual Congress on Healthcare Leadership) see and learn from many of these military leaders.

    The opening vignette in this chapter is based on a true story. Healthcare leaders in the armed forces do not work in a top-down, command-and-control environment. Obviously, a certain amount of discipline and authority exists in the military, but the dynamic is nothing like many believe. Military healthcare leaders have to cultivate a high trust level while developing the same competencies as civilian healthcare executives. My work with leaders in the Medical Service Corps, the Medical Corps, and the Army Nurse Corps over the past 35 years tells me they are exceptional leaders. I thank them and applaud their service, sacrifice, and dedication.

REFERENCES

Crandall, D. (ed). 2006. *Leadership Lessons from West Point*. San Francisco: Jossey-Bass.

Cuddy, A. 2015. *Presence: Bringing Your Boldest Self to Your Biggest Challenges*. New York: Little, Brown and Company.

Cuddy, A. J. C., M. Kohut, and J. Neffinger. 2013. "Connect, Then Lead." *Harvard Business Review*. Published July. https://hbr.org/2013/07/connect-then-lead.

Kotter, J. 1996. *Leading Change*. Boston: Harvard Business School Press.

Kouzes, J. M., and B. Z. Posner. 1993. *Credibility: How Leaders Gain and Lose It, Why People Demand It*. San Francisco: Jossey-Bass.

Lencioni, P. 2002. *The Five Dysfunctions of a Team: A Leadership Fable*. San Francisco: Jossey-Bass.

Office of News and Public Information. 2009. "Voluntary and Regulatory Measures Are Needed to Reduce Conflicts of Interest in Medical Research, Education, and Practice." The National Academies. Published April 28. www8.nationalacademies.org/onpinews/newsitem.aspx?RecordID=12598.

Robbins, S. P., and T. A. Judge. 2013. *Essentials of Organizational Behavior*, 12th ed. Upper Saddle River, NJ: Prentice Hall.

Rubenstein, D. 2016. Personal communication with author, May 15.

Schawbel, D. 2016. "Amy Cuddy: How Leaders Can Be More Present in the Workplace." *Forbes*. Published February 16. www.forbes.com/sites/danschawbel/2016/02/16/amy-cuddy-how-leaders-can-be-more-present-in-the-workplace/#4d39bef166ce.

Scholtes, P. R. 1998. *The Leader's Handbook: Making Things Happen, Getting Things Done.* New York: McGraw-Hill.

SUGGESTED READINGS

Anderson, C., and S. Brion. 2014. "Perspectives on Power in Organizations." *Annual Review of Organizational Psychology and Organizational Behavior* 1: 67–97.

Avolio, B., and W. L. Gardner. 2005. "Authentic Leadership Development: Getting to the Root of Positive Forms of Leadership." *Leadership Quarterly* 16 (3): 339–40.

Bobbio, A., and A. M. Manganelli. 2015. "Antecedents of Hospital Nurses' Intention to Leave the Organization: A Cross Sectional Survey." *International Journal of Nursing Studies* 52 (7): 1180–92.

McCabe, T. J., and S. Sambrook. 2014. "The Antecedents, Attributes and Consequences of Trust Among Nurses and Nurse Managers: A Concept Analysis." *International Journal of Nursing Studies* 51 (5): 815–27.

Nair, S. M., and R. Salleh. 2015. "Linking Performance Appraisal Justice, Trust, and Employee Engagement: A Conceptual Framework." *Procedia: Social and Behavioral Sciences* 211: 1155–62.

Pfeffer, J. 1992. *Managing with Power: Politics and Influence in Organizations.* Boston: Harvard Business School Press.

Swenson, S., G. Gorringe, J. Caviness, and D. Peters. 2016. "Leadership by Design: Intentional Organization Development of Physician Leaders." *Journal of Management Development* 35 (4): 549–70.

van der Werff, L., and F. Buckley. 2014. "Getting to Know You: A Longitudinal Examination of Trust Cues and Trust Development During Socialization." *Journal of Management.* Published July 24. http://jom.sagepub.com/content/early/2014/07/24/0149206314543475.abstract.

CHAPTER 16

Conflict Management

Although conflict can be uncomfortable, it is not unhealthy, nor is it necessarily bad. The question is not "How can people avoid conflict and eliminate change?" but rather "How can people manage conflict and produce positive change?"

—Peter G. Northouse (2016)

NEWLY HIRED JACK Lewis is a vice president of nursing clinical quality and education. Among his many responsibilities are nursing education and supervision of the clinical nurse specialists (CNSs). During his orientation, Jack rotated through various patient care units, talking with the managers and staff about his goals for improved patient safety and quality and a more comprehensive and coordinated nursing education program. Throughout his visits, he was well received by all staff. One week after his visit to surgery, he received the following e-mail from Margaret Strong, the vice president of surgical nursing. Margaret reports to Mike Volkman, the chief operations officer, and not to Lisa Apolinario, the chief nursing officer who is Jack's boss:

Jack,
I appreciate your enthusiasm for nursing quality and education. I must tell you that surgical nursing is different from the

rest of nursing at the hospital. Surgery does not have a need for your services. I have talked to Mike and Lisa, and it has been decided that the CNSs who work in surgery will now be under my direct supervision effective immediately. Please do not plan any nursing education or quality improvement programs for surgery because we intend to continue to use our own courses. Thank you for your attention to this matter.

Margaret

CONFLICT IS THE natural byproduct of the human thought process. It is present in us and is exacerbated by our interactions. The workplace, especially where decisions are made and implemented, hosts various kinds of conflict. How big a conflict becomes and how fast it spreads depend on the number of people involved, the situation's degree of difficulty, and the power structure in place.

Healthcare management is a breeding ground for conflict, as its issues span from operational to strategic and all points in between and even beyond. Such conflicts require leaders to be engineers of consent. That is, they must invite others to suggest solutions, guide that discussion, build consensus, and manage the discord that arises.

A conflict management guideline will help the leader and management team in this regard. Such a document, however, was shunned for years by many organizational leaders. They knew it was a critical instrument, but they offered myriad excuses for not creating one, including lack of time and few incidents of conflict. Fortunately, in 2009, The Joint Commission issued a mandate: All hospitals and health systems must develop and put into practice a guideline for managing conflict in leadership

> When engaging in conflict with peers, be careful not to allow your words or actions to cross into areas that might be perceived as unethical. In the heat of the moment, the lines between effective politicking and office sabotage can blur quickly, so leaders should have a mental checklist that they go through when they engage with a colleague.
>
> —Carson F. Dye and Brett D. Lee (2016)

teams. Recognizing that leadership conflicts can endanger human lives, The Joint Commission (2015, 106) states: "Conflict commonly occurs even in well-functioning hospitals and can be a productive means for positive change. However, conflict among leadership groups that is not managed effectively by the hospital . . . has the potential to threaten health care safety and quality. Hospitals need to manage such conflict so that health care safety and quality are protected. To do this, hospitals have a conflict management process in place."

HOW CONFLICT IS BENEFICIAL

Conflict is not fundamentally good or bad. After all, conflict represents our ability to reason, to work through a maze of possibilities and impossibilities. Also, it signifies the diversity of our perspectives, interests, and experiences. However, conflict can cause difficulty when not properly addressed.

In team functions, conflict also presents benefits, such as the following:

- *Ends complacency.* Conflict opens team members' eyes. They begin to see obstacles, inefficiencies, outdated practices, improprieties, and the like.
- *Starts dialogue.* Conflict almost always triggers a discussion—often heated and often generating more conflict. The once-quiet majority (or minority) then adds its voice to the conversation. Everyone really has something to say.
- *Activates a plan.* Conflict typically causes action; the action planned often is the solution to the conflict.
- *Forces participation.* The progression of conflict among team members often means that the conflicting parties will work together on the solution.

The ultimate problem with conflict is that it intimidates many people. Thus, it is seldom addressed—and inappropriately at that. Typically, minor conflicts—those that have no lasting implications—are ignored because they usually resolve themselves. However, over time, even minor conflicts (if persistent and repetitive) have the potential to turn major and corrupt and disrupt the team's performance and purpose.

THE CONCEPT IN PRACTICE

Following are strategies for preventing and responding to team conflicts.

Create a Conflict Management Policy

The first step toward conflict management is acknowledging that conflict inevitably occurs when intelligent, opinionated people converge. The second step is developing rules so that when a conflict does occur, all members can debate, deliberate, and compromise accordingly. These rules should be reviewed regularly by all members, and new members must be informed of their existence. Exhibit 16.1 is an example of conflict management guidelines.

Root Out the Potential Causes of Conflict

Meeting format and length, team size and composition, and member assignments and responsibilities are petri dishes for conflict. The leader should observe these areas for potential and hidden troubles that render the team ineffective. For example, if the team meets too often, team members are not given the time to do their work. Similarly, if vocal members dominate every team discussion, the rest of the group may harbor resentment for not having the chance

Exhibit 16.1 Conflict Management Guidelines

1. *Declare the conflict.* Not all discussions during group interaction are conflict oriented. When a struggle ensues, however, someone must inform everyone that a conflict has arisen so that proper procedures can be followed. Although this kind of statement may sound trite, it can become a powerful tool for managing conflict appropriately.

2. *Give the reason for the conflict.* Although disagreements and arguments are normal and necessary, they should not be initiated out of caprice or malice. Strife, hostility, and animosity must still be avoided at all cost, but if they do surface the reason (or reasons) for them must be stated.

3. *Clarify the issues of the conflict.* A neutral group member or one who is not directly embroiled in the conflict must be elected to clarify contentions and interpret ambiguities. All members must actively participate in the discussion or debate and specify in detail their issues. Although members are entitled to express their personal concerns or emotional responses, facts (not opinions) must govern the debate.

4. *Address one issue at a time.* To ensure appropriate and thoughtful consideration of all issues, only one issue at a time must be considered. Many people prefer to save their issues and raise them all during debates, but that practice should not be allowed or tolerated. All members should address their concerns as they occur.

5. *Require all members to participate in the debate.* No party in the dispute is allowed to "pull in his head" during the conflict. All members must give their opinion and not cower behind others on their side.

6. *Be fair.* Members must keep their "weapons" appropriate to the level of the fight. In other words, no personal attacks are allowed in a strictly professional discussion, and each party is given an opportunity to respond to accusations and defend itself.

7. *Declare that the conflict is over.* All members must know that the debate has ended and an outcome has been reached. The outcome agreement should be specifically defined so that no confusion, which could escalate into another conflict, will arise later.

to talk, which discourages their participation. See exhibit 16.2 for more causes of conflict.

The point here is that a leader can be more proactive in managing conflict if she knows where it usually starts.

Adopt a Format That Works for the Team

Team members should help establish a format for the meetings. This way, they are more apt to uphold it. For example, each meeting is run by a team member, who also creates the agenda, invites guests if needed, distributes necessary materials before the meeting, leads the discussions, and so on. No matter the format suggested, the leader should make every effort to adopt one that promotes involvement, reduces cynicism, and benefits the attendees.

Exhibit 16.2 Reasons for Conflict

- Incompatible personalities or value systems
- Overlapping or unclear job boundaries
- Competition for limited resources
- Inadequate communication
- Interdependent tasks (e.g., one person cannot complete his assignment until others have completed their work)
- Organizational complexity (i.e., the greater the decision-making layers and special requirements, the greater the conflict)
- Unreasonable or unclear policies, standards, or rules
- Unreasonable deadlines or extreme time pressure
- Collective and consensus decision making
- Unmet expectations
- Unresolved or suppressed tension

Source: Adapted from Kreitner and Kinicki (2012).

Practice Directspeak

Directspeak, a term I coined for speaking directly and clearly, is a straightforward manner of communicating without being insensitive. Directspeak does not work everywhere, but it thrives in team settings in which trust prevails, because every member of these teams knows that confrontations are never meant to be personal attacks. See exhibit 16.3 for a guide to Directspeak. CEOs or team leaders must be aware that some team members are uncomfortable with this technique, toe the line to avoid offending others, and are not active participants in debates. Conversely, some members are strong-willed and more verbal, which may intimidate the mild-mannered members. What results is another conflict: a personality conflict.

> Management teams whose members challenge one another's thinking develop a more complete understanding of the choices, create a richer range of options, and ultimately make the kinds of effective decisions necessary in today's competitive environments.
>
> —Kathleen Eisenhardt, Jean Kahwajy, and L. J. Bourgeois III (1997)

Exhibit 16.3 How to Practice Directspeak

Do	Don't
Speak with precision and clarity	Speak with vagueness and ambiguity
Make sure the debate takes place in the room	Allow the debate to take place in the hallway
Invite all questions	Make some questions off-limits
Keep discussion impersonal	Allow personal smears
Begin with the end in mind	Make us guess where you're going
Say something if you feel strongly about it	React strongly later in the conversation
Ask for clarification if needed	Assume or wait for a later time
When asked a question, answer it directly	Take the long way around to the "yes," "no," or "I don't know"

Prohibit Personal Attacks

Strong personalities (and hence opinions) can usher in conflict. One way to minimize personality-induced conflict is to keep the discussion focused on the issues, not the people. The leader should step in when inappropriate comments are introduced. Spirited debates are invigorating, especially if they do not include personal attacks. When team members veer off topic, the leader (e.g., CEO) could get up and jot down on the flip chart the goals of the discussion. His movement alone—not to mention that fact that he is pointing out the meeting's objectives—is often enough to rein in the chaos.

Choose a Collaborative Approach

As mentioned in chapter 14, the five usual reactions to conflict are as follows:

1. Avoid the other party and thus the conflict
2. Give in to the demands of the other party
3. Compete, with a goal to win
4. Compromise or strike a deal
5. Collaborate, with a goal to achieve

These responses illustrate the sink-or-swim mind-set among team members.

Avoidance is valid only when the conflict is too minor to merit full-time consideration—that is, when the problem will resolve itself without intervention. Giving in or surrendering is tied to the system of bartering favors (see chapter 15). Although well employed by teams, bartering is a temporary fix and could lead to more conflict if not executed appropriately. Competition, sometimes called *forcing*, creates an all-or-nothing environment in which team members do everything possible to defeat their perceived enemies. In this sense, team meetings become a personal battlefield where members show off their achievement to gain more power. Compromise, while democratic, stalls conflict resolution because it relies on too many people and too many variables.

Collaboration usually bests all other responses. It is a mature approach, not merely a reaction, to conflict that yields long-term benefits. The leader should verbalize her support of collaboration and put in place goals and activities that require inter-disciplinary partnerships.

A very popular research tool called the Thomas-Kilmann Conflict Mode Instrument (TKI) presents a solid model for understanding conflict. Essentially, it suggests that people's behavior when interacting stems from one of two basic dimensions—their desire to satisfy their own concerns (measured by their degree of personal assertiveness) or their willingness to satisfy the other person's concerns (measured by their degree of cooperativeness). Exhibit 16.4 shows this relationship.

> Teams must agree on how they will work together to accomplish their purpose and goals. Real team members always do equivalent amounts of real work beyond and between meetings where things are discussed and decided. Over time, a team's working approach incorporates a number of spoken or unspoken rules that govern contribution and membership.
>
> —Douglas K. Smith (1996)

The TKI suggests that five conflict styles emanate from this dynamic: competing (satisfying your own concerns), accommodating (sacrificing your concerns to meet the concerns of others), avoiding (ignoring the conflict), collaborating (finding a solution that is fully win–win for both parties), and compromising (finding a solution that is a partial win–win for both parties). Leaders can learn much about conflict by studying these concepts. Sample TKI assessments can be found on the Internet.

Visualize the End of the Conflict

Conflict has a beginning. That's the bad news. The good news is it also has an end. By visualizing the ideal outcomes of a conflict, the team is also generating ideas to prevent and manage it. For example, if the desired or visualized outcome is regular and relevant

Exhibit 16.4 Thomas-Kilmann Conflict Mode Instrument

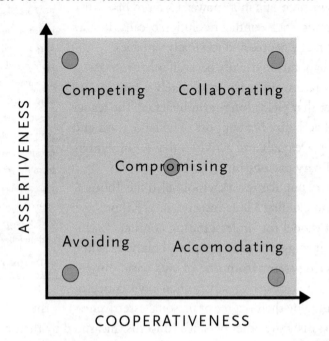

Source: Adapted from Thomas and Kilmann (2016). www.kilmanndiagnostics.com/overview-thomas-kilmann-conflict-mode-instrument-tki.

communication between physicians (through the chief medical officer) and the C-suite, then the team could work backward, analyzing the causes of the conflict, brainstorming practical solutions, developing action steps, and assigning responsibilities for implementing those steps. Although conflicts do end, the end still has to be closely monitored to ensure that the same conflicts do not resurface.

CONCLUSION

To a strong team, conflict is a temporary foe but a permanent ally. To a weak team, it is a predator. Regardless of its role, conflict is an inevitable occurrence in organizational life. Teams must understand that it is under their control.

Self-Evaluation Questions

❑ How does my team manage conflict? Is our approach working? If not, why not?

❑ What is my personal conflict management style? Is it working?

❑ Does my team suppress conflict? Why?

❑ Has my team established a conflict management policy? Was it developed for the team's sake, or to comply with requirements of The Joint Commission?

❑ How has conflict affected me personally?

Cases and Exercise
Case 16.1
Professor William Bligh, a retired ship captain, writes the following on the board:

- Power and influence
- Bigger is better
- Anger
- Emotional intelligence
- Bargaining
- Bullying
- You scratch my back and I'll scratch yours
- Scorekeeping

(continued)

(continued from previous page)

Then he addresses the class: "Write a ten-page paper about how each of these concepts contributes to team conflict. I expect to see your papers in two days. Class dismissed."

Give thought to what the students might prepare. How might the answers from a class of older, part-time students in a master's of health administration program be different from those given by people in a full-time residential program where most students are in their early twenties?

Consult the following books to gain a better understanding of team conflict:

Fisher, R., and W. L. Ury. 2011. *Getting to Yes: Negotiating Agreement Without Giving In*, 3rd ed. New York: Penguin.

Patterson, K., J. Grenny, R. McMillan, and A. Switzler. 2005. *Crucial Confrontations: Tools for Resolving Broken Promises, Violated Expectations, and Bad Behavior*. New York: McGraw-Hill.

Case 16.2

Jessica, Brianna, Ruth, and Zachary are assistant vice presidents in a large teaching hospital. Every month, they gather with their mentor, Dr. Lon Right, to talk about the challenges they face on the job and the trends in management and leadership. This month, they are discussing the book *Crucial Confrontations*.

> DR. RIGHT. On the basis of our reading, what should be the ultimate goal in resolving conflict?

JESSICA. To resolve the conflict and get compromise on the matter. Get the parties to meet halfway and then move on.

BRIANNA. I totally disagree. Compromising often means that you get poor results. Solving conflict does not mean you should give up on your key principles.

ZACHARY. I can see both sides. The real goal of conflict management, though, is to mount the debate but to do it in a respectful manner. Get the issue on the table, agree clearly on what the end goal is, and then hammer out the solution.

RUTH. In my view, practically all conflict is a classic power struggle. Human beings resolve these power struggles through fighting for their right to be heard. Compromises don't always happen, but what the book teaches us is how to negotiate with others so that we don't damage the relationships we worked hard to build.

Case 16.2 Questions

1. Is the ultimate goal of conflict management winning an argument, preserving a relationship, compromising on a solution, or all of these?

2. What lessons from this chapter and from *Crucial Confrontations* can be applied to your conflict management efforts?

Exercise 16.1

Read the vignette in the beginning of the chapter and answer the following questions:

(continued)

(continued from previous page)

- What kind of conflict is present in this situation?

- What are the short- and long-term effects of this conflict on the two nurse leaders involved, their chief executives, and the education of the CNSs?

- What should Jack's next step be?

- What organizational structure issues exist that gave rise to this conflict? How may they be resolved?

- The vignette illustrates an age-old story of strife between line and staff. What are some ways that these stresses can be avoided?

REFERENCES

Dye, C. F., and B. D. Lee. 2016. *The Healthcare Leader's Guide to Actions, Awareness, and Perception*, 3rd ed. Chicago: Health Administration Press.

Eisenhardt, K. M., J. L. Kahwajy, and L. J. Bourgeois, III. 1997. "How Management Teams Can Have a Good Fight." *Harvard Business Review* 75 (4): 77–85.

Joint Commission. 2015. *Hospital Accreditation Standards*. Oak Brook Terrace, IL: The Joint Commission.

Kreitner, R., and A. Kinicki. 2012. *Organizational Behavior*, 10th ed. Burr Ridge, IL: McGraw-Hill Education.

Northouse, P. G. 2016. *Leadership: Theory and Practice*, 7th ed. Los Angeles: SAGE Publications.

Smith, D. K. 1996. *Taking Charge of Change: 10 Principles for Managing People and Performance*. New York: Addison-Wesley.

Thomas, K. W., and R. H. Kilmann. 2016. "An Overview of the Thomas-Kilmann Conflict Mode Instrument (TKI)." Accessed May 22. www.kilmanndiagnostics.com/overview-thomas-kilmann-conflict-mode-instrument-tki.

SUGGESTED READINGS

Chiarchiaro, J., R. A. Schuster, N. C. Ernecoff, A. E. Barnato, R. M. Arnold, and D. B. White. 2015. "Developing a Simulation to Study Conflict in Intensive Care Units." *Annals of the American Thoracic Society* 12 (4): 526–32.

Johansen, M. L., and E. Cadmus. 2016. "Conflict Management Style, Supportive Work Environments and the Experience of Work Stress in Emergency Nurses." *Journal of Nursing Management* 24 (2): 211–18.

Johnson, S. L., D. M. Boutain, J. H. C. Tsai, R. Beaton, and A. B. de Castro. 2015. "An Exploration of Managers' Discourses of Workplace Bullying." *Nursing Forum* 50 (4): 265–73.

Kim, S., E. Buttrick, I. Bohannon, R. Fehr, E. Frans, and S. E. Shannon. 2016. "Conflict Narratives from the Health Care Frontline: A Conceptual Model." *Conflict Resolution Quarterly* 33 (3): 255–77.

Schaubhut, N. 2007. *Technical Brief for the Thomas-Kilmann Conflict Mode Instrument*. Psychometrics. Accessed May 22, 2016. www.psychometrics.com/wp-content/uploads/2015/02/tki-technical-brief.pdf.

Wong, C. A., P. Elliott-Miller, H. Laschinger, M. Cuddihy, R. M. Meyer, M. Keatings, C. Burnett, and N. Szudy. 2015. "Examining the Relationships Between Span of Control and Manager

Job and Unit Performance Outcomes." *Journal of Nursing Management* 23 (2): 156–68.

Yeung, D. Y., H. H. Fung, and D. Chan. 2015. "Managing Conflict at Work: Comparison Between Younger and Older Managerial Employees." *International Journal of Conflict Management* 26 (3): 342–65.

PART IV

EVALUATION

CHAPTER 17

Assessing Team Values

*For teams to be successful, the organizational
culture needs to support member involvement.*

—Peter G. Northouse (2016)

THE MESSAGE OF this book is simple: The leader and the team
(separately and together) must subscribe to a set of values that can
support and enhance effectiveness and success now and in the future.

What are your team values? Does your team discuss these values?
Are these values embedded in the norms and activities of the team?
What team behavior and practice will you change or improve to
live by these values?

This chapter explores the values that drive team functions and
performance. It guides you in assessing how well your leadership
team—specifically its members—upholds the team and other values.

KEY VALUES FOR ASSESSMENT

Team members should regularly assess the team's values. This activity reveals areas of deficiency and curtails harmful practices. Taplin,
Foster, and Shortell (2013, 280) state, "For leaders to help create and
support effective teams, they must know what conditions encourage

effective functioning of a particular type of team in a particular setting."

The following list, along with the questions posed after each item, may be used to start a values discussion with the team. Team members may compare and contrast their answers and then offer suggestions for improvement.

Competence

Basic competencies are expected of every leadership team. (For an extended list of leadership competencies, see Dye and Garman 2015.) Specifically, team members must possess a triumvirate of skill types—technical, decision making, and interpersonal. Each of these skills is critical for a leadership role, but together they strengthen the leader and make her a sustainable member of the team. The team member does not have to possess expert-level abilities, but she must be able to harness each skill at any time.

For example, if a team member has great technical acumen (e.g., finance, technology, business savvy) but lacks interpersonal skills, she may avoid opportunities to socialize with other team members, display behaviors that alienate her staff and other team members, fail to share or communicate information, and not participate in general discussions or team-building exercises. Similarly, if a team member has plenty of interpersonal charms but no decision-making instinct or technical abilities, he may not be able to perform the basic business responsibilities of a leader—let alone a team member.

> To engage people in strategies and create better business results, organizations require discussions that are authentic and real. Most companies and teams don't know how to have these conversations.
>
> —Jim Haudan (2008)

Ask yourself: Does the team value competence? Do members of my team possess a triumvirate of skills, at least? If not, what improvements are needed?

Awareness

It is helpful if team leaders understand the conditions that contribute to or enable team excellence.

—Peter G. Northouse (2016)

In an effective team, members are aware of each other's roles and responsibilities as well as the team's purpose, standards (or norms), and goals. Moreover, each member keeps abreast of current and future initiatives of the team. In this environment, all team members share information, discuss matters openly, and offer recommendations.

> **Ask yourself:** Are all team members aware of our collective purpose, goals, and norms as well as each other's roles and responsibilities? If not, what improvements are needed?

Active Participation

Awareness comes from active participation in all that the team does, including meeting discussions, planning activities, goals and standards development, decision making, and role assignments. Even when not all members are directly involved or needed in a team activity, cooperative members are still considered participants because they attend meetings, volunteer their time and talent, express and listen to opinions and ideas, give feedback, contribute to the camaraderie, and support collaboration.

Participation is crucial in attaining buy-in. That is, if team members are involved in any team activity from the start, they tend to commit to the initiative and encourage others to follow suit.

> **Ask yourself:** Do members of my team actively participate in our activities and initiatives? If not, what improvements are needed?

Cohesiveness

Team cohesiveness reduces personal animosity and organizational politics among members. It also increases the possibility that team goals will be achieved. Although cohesiveness presents several disadvantages, such as groupthink and low tolerance for change, it leads the way to cooperation and collaboration.

> **Ask yourself:** Is my team cohesive? If so, is my team aware of the danger of groupthink? If not, should we discuss it?

Commonality

A shared goal, values, or even profession is sometimes enough to bond people together. If the commonality is a shared goal, the effort put into achieving that objective is maximized, as everyone is working toward the same vision. Having commonality also means that team members may require less explanation and convincing about an initiative and the ensuing process. One negative aspect of commonality is that it could lead to the formation of cliques, which harm the cohesiveness of the team.

> **Ask yourself:** Does my team have a commonality? If so, how is it helpful? If not, what improvements are needed?

Commitment

When team members are committed (which is often brought about by cohesiveness and commonality), they work harder, set aside personal agendas, and contribute readily to team efforts. Simply put, committed members are highly engaged. This level of engagement generates thoughtful questions, creative and multifaceted solutions, and ambitious but feasible objectives. More important, the undertaking to which the members are committed results in desired outcomes.

> **Ask yourself:** Is my team committed to our purpose, goals, and tasks? If not, what improvements are needed?

Communication

Communication (including sharing of information and meeting discussions) enables the team to move forward. For work purposes, communication informs decision making, defines parameters (e.g., deadlines, goals, expectations, tasks), clarifies responsibilities, and prevents misunderstanding, to name a few functions. For interpersonal purposes, communication eases member interactions, assists with conflict resolution, and strengthens cohesiveness. Team communication—formal and informal, written and oral—should be regular, open, candid, and accurate.

> The use of dyads in leadership is a significant new topic for any healthcare leader hoping to adapt her organization to the clinical integration world. The subject is covered comprehensively in Kathleen Sanford, FACHE, and Stephen Moore's *Dyad Leadership in Healthcare: When One Plus One Is Greater Than Two* (2015). Sanford and Moore draw on their experiences creating clinical dyads to describe how this style of management can help healthcare organizations foster physician leadership—while managing the gaps in physician training—through collaboration with other managers. As of 2016, no other thorough treatments of this important leadership tool exist.

Ask yourself: How well do my team members communicate with one another? Does our communication produce desired outcomes? If not, what improvements are needed?

Independence Versus Interdependence

Interdependence can be likened to cohesiveness in that it is good, but it has its limits. In other words, an interdependent team is naturally collaborative. The members are supportive of each other, and they can rely on each other to fill in gaps in skills, for example.

Too much interdependence can strip the individual members of their independence, which is dangerous in healthcare delivery. For example, an interdependent team usually makes decisions as a unit. If one member is unexpectedly gone, the rest of the people on the team may not know what to do or may not be empowered to exercise their skills or authority. This indecision is counterproductive and does not forward the team's function. This example works for both administrative and clinical teams.

Ask yourself: How interdependent is my team? To what extent do my team members rely on each other for support and input in decision making? Are team members independent or empowered to make decisions? If not, what improvements are needed?

Camaraderie

Camaraderie is the goodwill among team members. It is the basis of active participation, cohesiveness, and communication. Team camaraderie develops when members spend time outside of the work context to get to know each other. Although it can form between members who have nothing in common, camaraderie is strongest when a commonality exists (and sometimes, being a member of the same team is common ground enough).

Ask yourself: Is there camaraderie among my team members? What do we do to maintain it?

High Energy

High energy makes the team more productive, creative, and participative. Energetic members anticipate team meetings and do not view them as a chore. Also, they are eager to receive new assignments and tasks, their minds already computing the details before they even begin.

Ask yourself: What is my team's energy level? Are my team members productive and eager? If not, what improvements are needed?

CONCLUSION

Every leadership team should periodically assess its values. If a team is productive and effective now (or "perfect"), imagine the even greater results it will achieve as it continues to lead by its values. Regular assessment of these values will help such a team sustain its success.

Ways to Boost Team Energy

- *Move a meeting to a different location, each time or occasionally.* A change of venue refreshes team member interests because it connotes a new beginning. Many retreats are effective solely because they take place outside of the office.

- *Celebrate team and individual accomplishments.* Festivities reverse moods positively, and good moods hike up energy levels.

- *Invite guest presenters.* Trained presenters inspire and rally people to act.

- *Take a break from routine.* This break does not need to be work related, but it should be fun and meaningful. For example, team members could volunteer at a homeless shelter or food pantry.

Self-Evaluation Question

❏ As a team member, what values do I espouse that may support or impede my team's function?

REFERENCES

Dye, C. F., and A. N. Garman. 2015. *Exceptional Leadership: 16 Critical Competencies for Healthcare Executives*, 2nd ed. Chicago: Health Administration Press.

Haudan, J. 2008. *The Art of Engagement: Bridging the Gap Between People and Possibilities.* New York: McGraw-Hill.

Morgeson, F. P., D. S. DeRue, and E. P. Karam. 2010. "Leadership in Teams: A Functional Approach to Understanding

Leadership Structures and Processes." *Journal of Management* 36 (1): 5–39.

Northouse, P. G. 2016. *Leadership: Theory and Practice*, 7th ed. Los Angeles: SAGE Publications.

Sanford, K., and S. Moore. 2015. *Dyad Leadership in Healthcare: When One Plus One Is Greater Than Two*. Philadelphia, PA: Wolters Kluwer.

Taplin, S. H., M. K. Foster, and S. M. Shortell. 2013. "Organizational Leadership for Building Effective Health Care Teams." *Annals of Family Medicine* 11 (3): 279–81.

SUGGESTED READINGS

Goleman, D. 2002. *Primal Leadership: Realizing the Power of Emotional Intelligence*. Boston: Harvard Business School Press.

Naylor, M. D., and E. T. Kurtzman. 2010. "The Role of Nurse Practitioners in Reinventing Primary Care." *Health Affairs* 29 (5): 893–99.

CHAPTER 18

Evaluating Team Effectiveness

Teamwork is an example of lateral decision making as opposed to the traditional vertical decision making that occurs in the organizational hierarchy based on rank or position in the organization.

—Peter G. Northouse (2016)

HOW DOES YOUR leadership team function? Is the team composition carefully put together, with an eye toward the organizational hierarchy? Are all team members involved in decision making? Are your meetings always, sometimes, or never necessary? Is the team bound to a set of protocols?

Garman and I argue that for teams to be effective, five critical activities are needed (Dye and Garman 2015):

1. Get the best people for team roles.
2. Develop an orientation toward a common vision and collective goals.
3. Develop trust among team members (as discussed in chapter 15).
4. Develop cohesiveness between team members.
5. Help team members productively work through the inevitable conflicts that come with group interaction.

The team's structure (size, hierarchy, membership) and primary activities (decision making, holding meetings, establishing team protocols) greatly affect its effectiveness, just as team values do. This chapter presents the components that a leadership team should assess on a regular basis.

TEAM STRUCTURE
Size

As mentioned in chapter 14, there is no ideal team size because every team has a different purpose, and this purpose dictates the number of members needed to make the team function well. However, there is such a thing as a team that is either too large or too small. Typically, a team that has 12 or more members is too large, while a team that has 4 or fewer members is too small. The problem with a large team is that decision making is slow, as too many people are involved in the process. With a small team, on the other hand, the expertise and experience of members may be limited, forcing the team to look outside for reinforcement and advice.

A team made up of 6 to 11 members works efficiently. Here, values (e.g., collaboration, cooperation) are more readily shared and learned, decisions are reached faster, tasks are more equally distributed, and conflicts are easier to spot and manage.

> **Ask yourself:** Is my team too large or too small? When was the last time my team assessed its size? What are the advantages and disadvantages of resizing my team?

Hierarchy

Although humility is the virtue that prevents people from boasting about their accomplishments and even compels them to say "titles don't mean anything," it is not the same virtue that commands people to be truthful. The importance of titles and status in the organization cannot be minimized. They are important, especially to high-ranking leaders (those in the C-suite).

A leader's title is not merely a short description of her job responsibilities; it bears prestige and influence. As such, it should be given its proper place on the team's hierarchy. For example, an executive vice president (VP) should be ranked higher than an assistant VP, and the two positions should not be given equal decision-making capabilities. One practice that fuels an imbalance of power among the team is granting undeserved titles either as an enticement for certain individuals to participate in an initiative or as a reward for an accomplishment that makes the team look good.

> All the empowered, motivated, teamed-up, self-directed, incentivized, accountable, reengineered, and reinvented people you can muster cannot compensate for a dysfunctional system. When the system is functioning well, these other things are just foofaraw. When the system is not functioning well, these things are still only empty, meaningless twaddle.
>
> —Peter R. Scholtes (1998)

Ask yourself: Does my team recognize and respect the hierarchy among our members? Do we inappropriately bestow titles?

Membership

Membership on the leadership team is a coveted and highly esteemed post. Unfortunately, appointment to this team (or even an invitation to attend its meetings) is often perceived by employees either as a privilege of being a leader or as a sign of cronyism. This perception is often justifiable, given that some departments and interests have a disproportionately large representation on the team and at its meetings (see exhibit 18.1 for examples).

To combat this perception, each membership appointment and invitation to meetings must be assessed according to practical, unbiased criteria, such as the following:

- The person's expertise, training, and skills
- The person's position and responsibilities
- The position's importance to the work and diversity of the team
- The position's potential contribution to the goals of the team
- Other work-related reasons for membership or attendance

Ask yourself: How is membership on my team viewed? As a privilege? As a reward? As a form of recognition? Does my team invite guests to our meetings, and how do they contribute to the discussion? Does my team follow established criteria for membership and meeting participation?

TEAM ACTIVITIES
Decision Making

Many teams are proficient in delaying (although not deliberately) decision making. Some teams discuss issues repeatedly but reach

---

Exhibit 18.1 Examples of an Imbalance of Power in a Leadership Team

- The public relations director is a member. She is in charge of disseminating organizational information to all staff.

- Both the senior VP of patient care services and the VP of nursing are members. Both have nursing backgrounds and thus skew clinical discussions toward nursing issues.

- Although not VPs, the director of human resources and the chief information officer are members.

- The director of the medical staff regularly attends team meetings, but he is not a member.

---

neither solution nor compromise. Other teams, meanwhile, are paralyzed by fear that any decision will create a conflict among team members. Yet decision making is a primary activity of a leadership team—an activity that cannot be delegated to another group or avoided without repercussions.

Often, the reason for this avoidance is the lack of a practical decision-making method. Specifically, basic components, such as the following, are missing:

> In the typical senior working group, individual roles and responsibilities are the primary focal points for performance results. There is not incremental performance expectation beyond that provided by individual executives working in their formal areas of responsibility.
>
> —Jon R. Katzenbach and Douglas K. Smith (1993)

- Facts and historical data about the issue at hand
- Brainstorming (for generating solutions and alternatives) and critical analysis tools and techniques (for examining ideas)
- Structured discussion method
- Well-defined goals and responsibilities
- Clear deadlines
- Trained leader or facilitator
- Participative members
- Time commitment

Ask yourself: Does my team employ a decision-making method? If not, how do we make decisions? Is my team known to delay or avoid making a decision, and what are the consequences of such an action? How do we handle disagreement or conflict about a decision? What can my team do to improve its decision-making skills?

Holding Meetings

Virtual meetings (which are more convenient) may eventually replace all traditional meetings, but even then team members will need to gather and discuss. They should. Meetings, if well planned and well run, enable the team to think together, something that an e-mail or a phone call, although more rapid, cannot provide. In addition, meetings are a key contributor to building camaraderie. Meeting attendees almost always have an opportunity before and after the meeting to socialize with each other.

The backlash against meetings points to poor planning. That is, people greatly dislike meetings because (1) they are time wasters, (2) they do not ensure anything will get accomplished, (3) they are scheduled one after another (or there are too many), and (4) they are a platform for ad nauseam discussions and show-offs.

Poor planning is the root cause of these complaints. This section offers strategies that can improve the major components of a meeting.

Necessity

Unfortunately, meetings have been so ingrained in the workplace that only few attendees question their purpose and relevance. The rest of us just show up. This conditioning is costly because while the leader is sitting in an unproductive and haphazard meeting, revenue-generating opportunities could be passing him by.

Here are two simple ways to determine if your attendance is necessary:

1. Review the minutes or notes from the last meeting and the agenda (if available) for the upcoming meeting.
2. Ask.

Ask yourself: Are all of our team meetings necessary? Have I questioned their relevance?

Objectives, Agendas, and Handouts

Objectives specify the purpose of the meeting. If a meeting is called just so the team can share information or updates but no discussions are expected, team members may request to send in their information (via e-mail perhaps) and be excused from attending. Although this option is not available to everyone, such as the meeting chair, it can free up time for those whose absence from the meeting will not make a difference.

Objectives are typically found on the meeting agenda. An agenda lists the items to be discussed in order of importance or according to the meeting format. Equipped with an agenda, team members can minimize digressions.

Handouts (e.g., financial statements, statistical reports, proposals) distributed before the meeting help attendees prepare their comments, questions, or suggestions. Fortunately, the protocol at most meetings now is that any item that comes with a handout will not be discussed if the materials are not disseminated ahead of time. Without this protocol, much of the meeting time is wasted on explaining background information.

Ask yourself: Does my team distribute an agenda with clear objectives? Who determines the objectives? Do our meetings follow the agenda? Are our meetings structured so as to prevent side conversations, multiple discussions, and other interruptions? Do we require and distribute handouts or preparatory material?

Roles and Norms

As mentioned in chapter 14, each team member must have a role to play (e.g., conscience, historian, devil's advocate). Such roles must conform to the norms (standards and expectations) of the team. For example, if the CEO is the chair, he must come prepared, come on time, come to stay, come to listen, come to participate, and come to ensure order during the meeting.

Ask yourself: What is my role, and does it abide by the norms that my team has set? What are my team's norms, and do we follow them closely? Do cliques or factions exist in my team? If so, do they have a different set of norms?

Time

Meetings are ravenous eaters of time. Flexible meetings are wasteful because they encourage too much deliberation and too little resolution. Although thoughtful discussions prevent risky undertakings, they are impractical in an environment pressured by constant change and quick fixes. The biggest time wasters are information-sharing meetings, which must not last longer than three hours. Although meetings in which strategies are developed and shaped must not have time limits, they should still be scheduled in advance and planned. Part of this planning is distributing a summary or minutes of the past meeting to refresh attendees. The minutes are also a great tool for initiating discussion.

> **Ask yourself:** How long do our meetings last? Do we have a regularly scheduled, time-limited meeting, or is it often flexible? Who keeps the minutes, and when are they distributed? Are the minutes detailed or vague, and are they useful for the next meeting?

Format

Generate creative ideas by making the meeting participatory.

This interactive format enhances the team's awareness of others' responsibilities and expertise, and it also displays team members' personalities, which could help develop commonality and camaraderie. Following are common (and often visual) approaches used during interactive discussions:

(continued from previous page)
and other components of team function? Who established them, and are they well known to and practiced by the team? What consequences are levied against those who disobey the rules?

6. *Conflict management.* What methods does the team employ to manage conflict? Is the team aware of the areas in which conflict may be introduced (e.g., decision making, discussions, power structure)?

- *Parking lot.* Innovative ideas not directly relevant to the current topic often emerge during a discussion. The parking lot is a way to save those ideas for later consideration.
- *Multivoting.* Multivoting is useful when the agenda lists too many items for discussion or consideration. Each team member is given a set number of votes to pick the issues (listed on a flip chart) she deems most important. All votes are cast confidentially to prevent political ramifications for the voters. The issues that receive the greatest number of votes remain on the agenda, and the rest are taken out. Multivoting is a democratic process that gives all members—especially the silent ones—a chance to be heard.
- *Affinity diagram.* This technique helps the team to organize and prioritize ideas and information. Using sticky notes, team members jot down data or suggestions and affix them to a flip chart. These notes are then arranged according to themes or categories. For example, "Use Twitter to create buzz about the new, green maternity ward," could be grouped under "marketing and communication."
- *Process mapping.* Process mapping alerts the team to the intricacies (i.e., responsibilities, tasks, measures, objectives) of a specific workflow. This technique is helpful when modifying an existing process and when creating a new one.

> High-performing teams are those with members whose skills, attitudes, and competencies enable them to achieve team goals. These team members set goals, make decisions, communicate, manage conflict, and solve problems in a supportive, trusting atmosphere in order to accomplish their objectives.
>
> —W. Gibb Dyer, Jeffrey H. Dyer, and William G. Dyer (2013)

Ask yourself: Are our meetings interactive and fun? If not, have we considered changing the format? What kind of participatory methods do we use?

Etiquette

Professional conduct must be expected in every professional setting. Distracting and rude behaviors (e.g., side conversations, flippant remarks) should not be tolerated during a meeting. Unfortunately, such behaviors (including the following examples) can be observed in leadership team meetings:

- Reading material unrelated to the team agenda to tune out an ongoing presentation
- Constantly stepping out to attend to a crisis or to take a break
- Constantly interrupting the facilitator or chair to ask a question, elucidate a point, complain, or argue
- Arriving late and unprepared
- Dominating the discussion and speaking out of turn
- Displaying dissent and impatience through body language, such as yawning, eye rolling, pounding on the table, and walking out
- Antagonizing a speaker or an idea with sarcastic comments and jokes
- Telling offensive (e.g., racist, sexist, elitist) jokes and anecdotes

The team, as a unit, should establish a code of conduct for meetings, post it in a visible setting or distribute it to all team members, and require all members to follow it. This code should include a clear statement about the consequences of not abiding by the rules. The team should also periodically discuss and evaluate the code.

Ask yourself: Has my team established etiquette guidelines? Generally, are my team members respectful? How does my team typically address inappropriate or distracting behaviors? What sanctions have been established for such cases?

Participation

Constant absence and nonparticipation may also fall under rude and distracting behavior. A team member who is not actively engaged impedes or slows down the team's work. In addition, conflicts of interest may arise when only part of the team is involved and represented in the decision making.

The team could draw quiet members into the discussion by using various methods, one of which is the nominal group technique (NGT). NGT's process is as follows:

1. Identify the problem.
2. Ask all members to offer at least one solution.
3. Write down, on a flip chart, all the ideas as they are suggested.
4. Discuss, clarify, and evaluate every idea on the list. Eliminate those that are repetitive or not feasible.
5. Compile a final list of solutions as agreed on by the team.
6. Ask all members to vote on each solution on the basis of its significance to their priorities. Each member gets one vote.
7. Rank the solutions according to the number of votes received.
8. Select the solution that garnered the top spot.

Ask yourself: How engaged are my team members? Does my team encourage everyone to participate? What kind of tools does my team use to support an all-member discussion?

Wrap-Up

End the meeting right. Many meetings last so long that, by the end, participants are so eager to leave that they fail to hear the last minutes of the discussion. The final minutes of any meeting should be the strongest because at this time the leader can rally support for the issues discussed and motivate the team to follow through. The team leader must conclude the meeting by providing a short summary (one or two sentences) of the issues discussed, the responsibilities assigned, and the steps that need to be taken before the next meeting.

> **Ask yourself:** How does my team end our meetings? Do members leave exhausted and overwhelmed with too much information? How do we remind members of the decisions made and the next steps?

Establishing Team Protocols

All team members should be involved in developing the protocols that govern its behaviors, interactions, activities, decisions, and all other dealings. Equal participation by all members ensures that the protocols are not just created but also obeyed.

Following is an example of a decision-making protocol established by the entire team.

1. *Decisions must be made by all members, not just by a subset.*
    Because some teams are too large, their leaders rely on
    a subgroup to deliberate on issues and make decisions.
    As a result, members outside of this subset may feel
    disrespected and could start a conflict. Conversely,
    members of the subgroup may feel arrogant and superior
    to the rest of the team. Although using a small group is a
    practical alternative to a lengthy all-member deliberation,
    it can harm team cohesiveness. If decisions must be made
    by a subset, the reasons must be explained to and discussed

by the entire team. This way, everyone is aware of the intentions, and a rift is less likely to develop.

2. *A decision-making process must be determined for the issue on hand.* Will a vote be taken? If so, will the decision be determined by a majority? Are some members' votes given more weight than others'? By discussing the process in depth, the team can avoid the Abilene paradox: A family made a long trip to Abilene, simply because one person suggested the location and the others believed that everyone agreed. As the family members returned from Abilene, they discovered that none of them had wanted to go to Abilene in the first place.

3. *Divergent or nontraditional ideas must not be discouraged.* Unique perspectives can strengthen decision making, introducing innovative concepts, problems, and consequences that the team may not have considered before.

4. *Team member expertise should not cause an imbalanced decision.* Teams have the tendency to allow clinical decisions to be guided solely by the chief nursing officer or the chief medical officer. Members without such training can also offer meaningful and creative approaches.

5. *Proper decorum and courtesy must always be practiced.* Respect and honor in debate and deliberation are essential to effective team outcomes.

CONCLUSION

Inefficiencies can easily creep into the smallest details of a team. Regular monitoring and evaluation ensure that the structure and activities of the team still function in its favor. After all, an inefficient team cannot produce a successful outcome, let alone sustain itself. See appendixes C and D for leadership team evaluation tools.

Self-Evaluation Questions

❑ What is the composition of my team? Does the membership evenly represent the major areas in the organization?

❑ How are our team meetings conducted? Do we abide by certain rules of conduct during the meeting?

❑ What is our decision-making process? Are my team members involved in discussions?

❑ Has my team established team protocols? Do we follow these protocols?

Exercises

According to an excellent article by Reader and colleagues (2009), there is a growing literature on the relationship between teamwork and patient outcomes in intensive care, providing new insights into the skills required for effective team performance. Review the article with other clinical leaders and determine what specific factors contained in the article might enhance team effectiveness. The article can be found at http://eprints.lse.ac.uk/29082/1/Developing_a_ team_performance_framework_for_the_intensive_care_ unit_(LSERO).pdf.

Geisinger Health System uses various criteria to target specific care models for redesign: those provider services with the largest impact by patient population or resource consumption, those with the greatest amount of unjustified variation, those with evidence-based or consensus-derived best practices and readily available outcome metrics, those with the most interest from clinical champions or consumers, or those with observed outcomes farthest from expected performance. Review Paulus, Davis, and Steele (2008) to find evidence of strong team structure in the Geisinger organization and its approach-to-care models. The article can be found at http://content.healthaffairs.org/content/27/5/1235.long.

REFERENCES

Dye, C. F., and A. N. Garman. 2015. *Exceptional Leadership: 16 Critical Competencies for Healthcare Executives*, 2nd ed. Chicago: Health Administration Press.

Dyer, W. G. Jr., J. H. Dyer, and W. G. Dyer. 2013. *Team Building: Proven Strategies for Improving Team Performance*, 5th ed. San Francisco: Jossey-Bass.

Katzenbach, J. R., and D. K. Smith. 1993. *The Wisdom of Teams: Creating the High-Performance Organization*. Boston: Harvard Business School Press.

Northouse, P. G. 2016. *Leadership: Theory and Practice*, 7th ed. Los Angeles: SAGE Publications.

Paulus, R. A., K. Davis, and G. D. Steele. 2008. "Continuous Innovation in Health Care: Implications of the Geisinger Experience." *Health Affairs* 27 (5): 1235–45.

Reader, T. W., R. Flin, K. Mearns, and B. H. Cuthbertson. 2009. "Developing a Team Performance Framework for the Intensive Care Unit." *Critical Care Medicine* 37 (5): 1787–93.

Scholtes, P. R. 1998. *The Leader's Handbook: Making Things Happen, Getting Things Done*. New York: McGraw-Hill.

SUGGESTED READINGS

Collins, C. G., C. B. Gibson, N. R. Quigley, and S. K. Parker. 2016. "Unpacking Team Dynamics with Growth Modeling: An Approach to Test, Refine, and Integrate Theory." *Organizational Psychology Review* 6 (1): 63–91.

Friedrich, T. L., J. A. Griffith, and M. D. Mumford. 2016. "Collective Leadership Behaviors: Evaluating the Leader, Team Network, and Problem Situation Characteristics That Influence Their Use." *Leadership Quarterly* 27 (2): 312–33.

Günzel-Jensen, F., A. K. Jain, and A. M. Kjeldsen. 2016. "Distributed Leadership in Health Care: The Role of Formal Leadership Styles and Organizational Efficacy." *Leadership*. Published May 12. http://lea.sagepub.com/content/early/2016/05/11/1742715016646441.abstract.

Hu, J., and R. C. Liden. 2015. "Making a Difference in the Teamwork: Linking Team Prosocial Motivation to Team Processes and Effectiveness." *Academy of Management Journal* 58 (4): 1102–27.

Reader, T. W., R. Flin, and B. H. Cuthbertson. 2011. "Team Leadership in the Intensive Care Unit: The Perspective of Specialists." *Critical Care Medicine* 39 (7): 1683–91.

Whittaker, G., H. Abboudi, M. S. Khan, P. Dasgupta, and K. Ahmed. 2015. "Teamwork Assessment Tools in Modern Surgical Practice: A Systematic Review." *Surgery Research and Practice*. Published September 30. http://www.hindawi.com/journals/srp/2015/494827/.

CHAPTER 19

Self-Evaluation at All Career Stages

Navigating effectively through life, creating a meaningful purpose in it, and ultimately, reflecting yourself, requires an organized perspective on life's structure.

—Michael P. McNally (2015)

TASHA RHONA, a search consultant, and her close friend Rebecca Boling-Rodriguez are on the phone regarding a recent job disappointment.

REBECCA. The search consultant just called to tell me I didn't get the CEO job. I have no idea why. I pushed him to give more details but he said it was close, but there was nothing I could have done to change the outcome. Apparently, I didn't make any mistakes in the interview process. Frankly, I have the experience and the skills. My interviews with the physicians went very well, or so I thought. In fact, two doctors approached me after the medical executive committee interview just to say they were looking forward to working with me. At the final interview, which felt like a welcome-to-the-club dinner meeting, the board chair and vice chair asked if I could think of any areas I needed special help or guidance with . . .

TASHA. How did you answer that?

REBECCA. With a no! What else am I supposed to say?

TASHA. Let's calm down here. In your 20-plus-year career, this was the first time you actually competed in a job search. You found your previous jobs via individuals with whom you had worked before. How could you have really known how to prepare for an interview? I can't tell you why they passed on hiring you, but I can tell you what they might have been looking for. Are you ready to hear that?

REBECCA. I have a feeling you'll tell me anyway.

TASHA. When was the last time you did a self-evaluation of your skills, your style, your values—the whole nine yards?

REBECCA. Why? Is that important?

VALUES-DRIVEN LEADERS are self-assessors. They understand that they cannot expect others to speak, think, and act according to principles if they do not demand the same things of themselves. Thus, these leaders study their own moves and thought processes, with the dual intention of personal improvement and professional achievement.

All leaders—early, mid-, and late careerists—can benefit from evaluating their performance or practice in various areas related to their respective career stages.

ALL CAREERISTS
Personal Mission Statement

A personal mission statement is the road map of any careerist, pointing to the desired destination and preventing the person from veering off course. This statement should answer the following questions:

- What is my purpose in life?
- What is my ultimate personal goal?
- What is my ultimate professional goal?
- What do I enjoy doing most?
- How and where do I make the most impact?
- How would I like my obituary to read? (Although morbid, this question forces you to think about your legacy.)

Writing this statement is daunting, taxing, frustrating, and awkward at first, but this tension eases after several drafts. Exhibit 19.1 provides examples of personal mission statements.

Reviewing the statement after a certain time is beneficial. Doing so will ensure that the document (1) is kept alive through daily deeds and words and (2) is revised to reflect the leader's values and goals. After several years, the statement can serve as a reminder of accomplishments and shortcomings. Some seasoned leaders have saved the mission statements they wrote when they were new to the field. One executive pulls out his old mission statements and self-evaluation notes annually. Revisiting them helps him find the "true north" of his personal life and career.

Ask yourself: Have I written a personal mission statement?

Personal and Professional Style

The Kuder Career Assessment or the Strong Interest Inventory are among the most commonly used tools for assessing career interests

Exhibit 19.1 Sample Personal Mission Statements

Sample 1

My faith and my family are the most important things in my life. I want to be remembered by my family as a loving spouse and a caring parent. I want my children to remember that I did do an effective job of balancing work and home. I want my spouse to be comfortable with my desire to make a difference in healthcare.

I will end up compromising these values if I take a bigger, better job with more prestige. I do not want to do this. Therefore, I must be cautious in being tempted by these kinds of jobs. I will enjoy serving in an organization where I can make a personal impact without neglecting my children and spouse.

Although I want to be a CEO, I understand that the trade-off with my family is not worth that price. So, I will try to serve my CEO so effectively that he will include me in more of his decision making and give me greater authority, and I will gain greater fulfillment. This will give me much of the satisfaction typically enjoyed by CEOs.

I will try to work in organizations that respect and support work/family balance. I will try to show this same respect for my division managers.

At the end of my life, I would like to be remembered as a person who was effective in balancing both family and career and one who did not allow work and career to take over.

Sample 2

I entered healthcare to serve others. As a clinician, I studied the art and science of healing. I want to keep this healing mission the central focus of my working life. I want others to know me as a person who always puts patients first. I will be a good steward of the skills given me and will work to get others around me to develop and sustain the passion for patient care that I possess.

I want to work in organizations that put missions first and margin second. I do not want to be affiliated with organizations that are not committed to high quality. I do not want to work in the for-profit health sector.

---

and proclivities. Other assessments provide insight into personal and professional styles and behaviors. Validated instruments such as the Hogan Personality Inventory; the Hogan Development Survey; and the Hogan Motives, Values, and Preferences Inventory provide in-depth insight into personality as it relates to the workplace. These inventory tools are applicable to the skills and styles expected of workers today, and they reflect the leadership competency systems that many organizations have begun to develop. Search consultant firms also employ assessment instruments to evaluate candidates.

Ask yourself: Am I aware of my personal and professional style? Do I use assessment tools, or do I rely on feedback alone?

Values

Constant review of values is imperative, as they affect priorities, behaviors, mind-set, and performance. Team or executive retreats, performance reviews, self-reflection exercises, and mentor meetings are forums for thinking about and discussing these values.

Unfortunately, stories about senior executives who have committed unethical acts have dominated the news in recent years. Such incidents exemplify that (1) no one is immune to the seductive power of high office and (2) many careerists—from new to veteran—verbally support great values but do not understand how to live those values or why they must do so.

Especially at senior management levels—at which increases in revenues, market share, and physician and customer satisfaction rates are the primary focus—values-based concepts tend to be viewed as window dressing.

Personal values drive many professional values. In this way, a deficiency in one is a deficiency in another. For example, a careerist who values self-interest tends to form or join a clique, sabotage cohesiveness and collaboration, and refrain from participating in initiatives that do not directly benefit him.

Ask yourself: What are my values? Are they aligned with those of my organization? If not, what is the difference, and is it hurting my chances of achieving my goals?

Continuing Education

Education should not stop with the completion of a graduate degree. In fact, such a degree is only an entrance ticket. Learning should be a lifelong pursuit because it makes the careerist more marketable, more in touch with current trends and practices, and more able to overcome challenges. Continuing education (both degree and nondegree programs) is offered by various entities, including professional associations, public agencies, private companies, and colleges and universities. Many such offerings are designed for working adults, as evinced by the proliferation of webinars, distance learning, night and weekend classes, and accelerated programs. The most accessible and inexpensive forms of learning are reading healthcare-related publications and discussing trends with colleagues.

> **Ask yourself:** How do I keep up with changes in healthcare, in the management field, and in my role? What can I do to expand my knowledge and skill base? Is my organization supportive of continuing education? If not, what other avenues of learning may I explore?

EARLY CAREERISTS
Mentor Relationship

An early healthcare careerist undoubtedly has a lot to learn. Who better to serve as teacher than a practicing healthcare leader? Graduate health administration curricula and professional management courses put much emphasis on the technical (including financial), administrative, and human resources aspects of leadership, but they often fail to cover behavior and ethics standards. A mentor can fill in for the new careerist the gaps that exist between education and practice, including interpersonal expectations. In addition, a mentor can introduce the new careerist to resources, provide advice and insight, clarify nuances, serve as a sounding board, and urge improvement.

> The secret of joy in work is contained in one word—excellence. To know how to do something well is to enjoy it.
>
> —Pearl S. Buck (1964)

Ask yourself: Do I have a mentor? What kind of relationship do I have with my mentor? Is this mentoring relationship beneficial to my career growth? If not, how may I improve it?

The Unexpected

Everything will be unexpected to the new careerist, especially in a fast-changing field such as healthcare. Preparation is the best response to the unexpected. It makes the person think quickly and creatively, retain interest and focus, and be less intimidated by the unknown. For example, an early careerist is far less reluctant to try an untested, risky idea if she has done her research, spoken with experts and other experienced staff, weighed the pros and cons, designed a backup and response plan, and communicated the information she has with her supervisees. This way, if the idea develops an unexpected glitch later on, the glitch will not cause a major disturbance for those involved.

Ask yourself: How well do I prepare for any activity? How do I respond to the unexpected?

Strengths and Weaknesses

An early careerist must be aware of his abilities and limitations, as this knowledge puts him in control of what can be enhanced, what can be mastered, and what can be delegated (although this option only works for nonrequired responsibilities such as volunteering on a team). For example, if the person knows he is not good with numbers, he can attend budgeting and finance classes, ask others for help in understanding the concepts, and seek opportunities for practicing or applying the skill. Awareness of a personal limitation humbles a person, but it also serves as an impetus for improvement.

Early careerists can benefit from knowing what their leaders expect. One CEO distributes the following list of knowledge, skills, and abilities she demands from her team:

- Concise communication
- Focus on results
- Listening skills
- Strategic thinking
- Consistent and appropriate behavior
- Drive and initiative
- Persuasion
- Customer and team orientation

Ask yourself: What are my strengths and weaknesses? Am I committed to improving and mastering my skills? Do I understand the perils of my weaknesses?

Broad Perspective

Many early careerists tend to focus on only one organizational function—strategic planning, financial analysis, operations, human resources, or some other specialty. Although this practice enables the careerist to master a certain discipline, it curbs creativity and narrows perspective. During the first years, the early careerist should be a generalist, learning all the functions and their interrelationships. An early careerist is expected to ask questions and listen intently. Everyone else feels obliged to share his knowledge and contribute to the early careerist's development. Nobody loses in this type of exchange.

Ask yourself: Do I shadow, ask questions of, and forge relationships with people with diverse knowledge and specialties? How much do I know about the inner workings of my job and others' jobs? How may I widen my understanding and perspective?

Organizational Politics

Early careerists are primarily focused on gaining project experience. As such, they tend to be oblivious to the political undercurrents surrounding them. These power struggles are often common knowledge among staff, who suffer the consequences, such as red tape, slow decision making, and multiple layers of approval. The early careerist should pay attention to signs of conflict and political upheaval, such as the following:

- Sudden departure of a well-liked, high-performing leader
- Distribution of multiple memos with divergent messages
- Side negotiations and secret campaigns
- Frequent "special" and closed-door meetings
- Increased backroom gossiping and theorizing
- Sudden cuts in budget, staff, and other resources
- Disruptions of routine
- Diminished morale
- Hierarchical or structural changes

Ask yourself: Am I aware of the political nuances in my organization? How do I find out about them?

Diligence

For an early careerist, every assignment is a test of skills, patience, persistence, and potential. Thus, the careerist must validate, double-check, corroborate, proofread, and reference every piece of information, as any errors and omissions can be viewed as the result of sloppy work. This diligence helps the careerist develop great habits, which are the root of effective performance.

Ask yourself: Is my work meticulous? If not, what can I do to improve?

Job Opportunities

Some early careerists spend five to six years in their first jobs without considering (or experiencing) a promotion, a lateral move to a different department, or a position in another organization. Part of the reason may be loyalty or complacency, but more often than not the reason is fear. At this early stage, careerists should only fear stagnation and burnout, not the possibility of a job opportunity.

Staying in one place for a long time is admirable; in fact, many successful leaders retire from the same organizations that originally hired them. However, today's healthcare environment thrives on change and newness, demanding its leaders to follow suit.

One way to pursue change (and prevent burnout) is to apply for job opportunities. This process, including interviewing, enables the careerist to tout her strengths, assess her weaknesses, articulate her goals, discover her earning and career potentials, learn about the job market, and interact with professionals in another workplace. In addition, the process sharpens the careerist's communication and negotiation skills and presents a fresh perspective.

Behold the turtle. He only makes progress when he sticks his neck out.

—James Bryant Conant (quoted in Hershberg 1993)

Ask yourself: How long ago did I apply for another job inside or outside my organization? Am I confident enough of my knowledge, skills, and abilities to pursue a promotion, a lateral move, or a job opening in a different institution? Do I think the application process (even if I don't intend to leave my job) is beneficial or harmful to my career growth, and why?

MIDCAREERISTS
Complementary Work and Home Life

"Busy" is the most succinct description of a midcareerist's workday, which can stretch for more than 14 hours at times. These long days, not to mention occasional weekend events, wreak havoc on personal time and relationships.

The tug of war between personal and professional life is a stressor faced by most, if not all, midcareerists. Although some are skilled at balancing these pursuits, many others struggle, leading to bad tendencies such as impatience, intolerance, arrogance, selfishness, and negative attitudes.

> **Ask yourself:** What can I do to live a balanced life? How is the imbalance in my life affecting my work, my relationships, and my future goals? To whom can I turn for help in this regard?

360-Degree Feedback

The 360-degree feedback instrument is the surest way to obtain frank comments from an array of people. The main reason for this is that the tool ensures confidentiality to participants, taking away the commenters' fear of reprisal. This tool, and similar feedback tools, is helpful to the midcareerist's development because the assessments come from those who work directly or have regular contact with the person. In addition, the tool evaluates a broad aspect of the careerist's performance.

Ask yourself: How often do I get feedback, and what tool do I use? Is the feedback I receive constructive or destructive? Do I promote the use of feedback to effect positive change? If not, why?

Networking

Networking breeds innovative ideas and fresh perspectives. Expanding their professional networks is most beneficial to midcareerists because at this stage they have been in the field long enough to have repeatedly tried the same strategies but not long enough to have become cynical about novel approaches. In addition, networking gives midcareerists another source of data and information, feedback, recommendations, and advice—all of which are essential to the work they do.

Ask yourself: What networking opportunities do I pursue? In what ways are they helpful?

Mentoring and Teaching Opportunities

Mentoring is beneficial to both parties involved. It allows the mentor to

- contribute to someone else's career development and growth;
- share insights into the implicit, unwritten, and unspoken rules of organizational life;
- offer advice on professional decisions that have the potential to turn into mistakes with long-lasting consequences;
- celebrate someone else's victories and provide counsel and comfort in that person's defeats;

- gain satisfaction and pride from being a vital resource, an advocate, a confidant, and a friend; and
- give back to (and do one's part for) the healthcare community.

The questions that a protégé poses can also prompt the mentor to reevaluate her own career path or choices. For example, one former CEO admits that she returned to being a chief operations officer after her protégé asked if she liked what she was doing. This question made the former CEO realize that she missed running day-to-day operations and the enjoyment she gained from that role.

Mentoring is fundamentally equal to teaching. Teaching, however, is structured, abides by rigid schedules, and requires much preparation. Practitioners are valuable additions to the faculty of any graduate program in health services administration because they strengthen the credibility of these programs. Many students prefer to learn from teachers who have field experience and who have applied (or created) methodologies explored in textbooks and other course materials. More important, students gain much insight from teachers who have actually failed and succeeded at making real-world, organization-wide decisions.

Teaching provides ample rewards for midcareer practitioners, including the following:

- Opportunities to learn about (or at least become familiar with) new trends, forecasts, best practices, general and specific concerns, and public opinions—both inside and outside the field
- Opportunities for self-reflection, values reassessment, and reevaluation of career choices
- Forums for discussing healthcare-related news, history, customers, operational challenges, strategic approaches, and similar topics

- Regular lessons in humility, open-mindedness, diverse perspectives and expectations, relationships, and values

Both mentoring and teaching enhance the mid-careerist's performance levels, preparing him for his next role.

Ask yourself: Am I a mentor or a teacher? If so, what advantages does each role present? If not, have I considered mentoring and teaching opportunities? Do I have a mentor or teacher who has been part of my growth?

LATE CAREERISTS
Retirement Planning

For active and busy late careerists, thinking about retirement can be traumatic for several reasons. First, their level of control will diminish. Second, the pace of their everyday lives will slow down. Third, the number of their associates will dwindle. Fourth, and most important, their sense of productivity and contribution will shrink. Regardless of such trepidations, retirement is inevitable and thus must be faced accordingly.

The late careerist must develop clear plans (for home and work purposes) for her departure and communicate those plans with her family and staff. Financial preparation is imperative, but it is not the sole element of a robust retirement plan, which should include a next-career transition plan.

The plans of some retired CEOs include the following elements:

Further Development Opportunities
The American College of Healthcare Executives provides extensive career services and support. Its online service, CareerEDGE, is a unique, interactive, comprehensive tool for planning and managing a career. Additional resources can be found at www.ache.org/newclub/career/career_development.cfm.

- A personal mission statement for the retirement years
- A phased plan for the next, less-rigorous occupation, such as being an instructor

Note that retirement planning is markedly different from succession planning. The latter is a structured, multilevel development process, while the former is a personal transition exercise.

> **My Creed**
>
> To have no secret place wherein
> I stoop unseen to shame or sin;
> To be the same when I'm alone
> As when my every deed is known;
> To live undaunted, unafraid
> Of any step that I have made;
> To be without pretense or sham,
> Exactly what men think I am.
>
> —Edgar Guest (1911)

Ask yourself: How am I preparing—intellectually, financially, physically, socially, and emotionally—for my retirement? Are my family and staff aware of my plans?

Attitude Toward Younger Colleagues and Aspiring Leaders

Some late careerists question the values (including commitment) and contributions of "today's generation," regarding young workers with cynicism and skepticism. This negative attitude runs counter to the values espoused by the late careerist and harms team morale. Hearing it is also offensive, even when said in jest. Seasoned leaders have accomplished too much to tarnish their reputation by making petty remarks.

Ask yourself: How do I regard the younger generation? Am I welcoming, or am I curmudgeonly? How do my colleagues respond to this attitude, and how are they affected?

Self-Tributes

Self-tributes are a documentation of not only the late careerist's achievements but also the positive changes to the organization, the community, and the lives of many people. Writing this tribute is not an exercise in egomania; rather, it is an exercise in self-affirmation—that is, it serves as a reminder that your personal sacrifices eased others' hardships, that you instituted improvements that saved lives and livelihood, or that your tireless advocacy and support led to progress in the community and the organization. After all, no one knows all the good that has been done better than the person who made it happen.

Ask yourself: What will people remember about me? Have I written a self-tribute? If not, what will I include in this document?

CONCLUSION

Finding time for self-assessment is more easily said than done. But doing so is not impossible, especially when a strong commitment to improvement exists. Self-evaluation and self-reflection are routine practice for successful leaders because they understand that even the most ideal people can be "consistently inconsistent"—that is, everyone falls victim to saying one thing but doing another. If we are not aware of this tendency, we cannot begin to remedy it. This book offers not only a detailed explanation of this tendency but also a strong remedy.

Self-Evaluation Questions

❑ Have I ever formally, using assessment tools, evaluated my leadership successes and failures?

❑ How well do I live by my values? Do I expect those around me to live by their values?

❑ What is my legacy?

REFERENCES

Buck, P. S. 1964. *The Joy of Children*. New York: J. Day.

Covey, S. R. 1990. *The Seven Habits of Highly Effective People: Powerful Lessons in Personal Change*. New York: Fireside Press.

Guest, E. A. 1911. *Just Glad Things*. Detroit.

Hershberg, J. G. 1993. *James B. Conant: Harvard to Hiroshima and the Making of the Nuclear Age*. New York: Knopf.

McNally, M. P. 2015. *Reflect Yourself: Exploring, Assessing, Understanding, and Improving Your Life*. Tucson, AZ: Wheatmark Publishing.

Shaw, G. B. 1906. *Mrs. Warren's Profession: A Play in Four Acts*. London: Archibald Constable and Co.

ACADEMIC PERSPECTIVES

CHAPTER 20

Maximizing Values-Based Leader Effectiveness

Jared D. Lock, PhD

THIS BOOK ASSERTS that leaders who understand, live within, and perform according to their values are personally and professionally successful. For the first edition of this book, the author asked me to write a chapter that linked this argument with strong empirical support. At the time, little was known about leadership in healthcare, and virtually no models of values effectiveness had been established. Today, more than a decade later, although healthcare executives are more aware of the connection between values and success, relevant literature in this area is still in short supply, and some studies (not empirical research) are poor in quality.

The reason I find some of these studies deficient is threefold. First, they were sponsored by private interests (e.g., assessment tool publishers, credentialing firms) to market their own products and thus are reductionist in nature; that is, they boil down this comprehensive concept of leadership to a short list of characteristics and offer no explanations about the drivers of success. Second, they are nothing more than personality surveys, which depend on subjective opinions and personal preferences rather than on evidence. Third, they present no unified or practical approach to understanding how a leader's values affect organizational success. As a result, such research fails to provide true measures of leadership values and effectiveness.

This chapter presents a framework—the whole-person model—for understanding leader effectiveness in the context of values. In addition, the chapter reviews findings from empirical research that support the clear connection between leadership values and high performance. It is interesting to note that, though the referenced research is not particularly new (some might say outdated), current reviews of the state of the field indicate little progression in the past 20 years (e.g., Effron 2014).

REVIEW OF THE LITERATURE: DEFINING LEADER EFFECTIVENESS

This section summarizes research findings regarding leadership performance—specifically, its outputs (effectiveness) and inputs (values and characteristics).

Most healthcare organizations consider financial performance to be the number one indicator of a leader's effectiveness. However, financial results do not identify what the leader did, why the leader did it, or what the leader could have done better.

Some studies define effectiveness as a *sustained* financial performance (e.g., more than 15 years) as compared with the competition. Organizations with sustained performance, the literature shows, have leaders who can influence the culture, impart value systems on others, and get others to follow those values (Hogan and Blake 1996). Specifically, these leaders do the following:

- Identify with and work in organizations that uphold the same goals and values as they do. With this kind of match, the leaders can easily motivate subordinates to perform according to their values (Borman and Motowidlo 1993; Guzzo and Shea 1992; Manz and Sims 1987).

- Control which goals are pursued in their organizations (Kouzes and Posner 2002).
- Change the value system (both positive and negative) of their organizations over time (Schneider 1987).

Research has also found the following:

- Leader values that are productive and in line with the organization's direction result in successful outcomes (Lock and Thomas 1998).
- Team counterproductivity is linked to a discrepancy between the leader's and the organization's value systems (Hackman 1987).

MEASURING LEADER PERFORMANCE: THE WHOLE-PERSON APPROACH

Research in this field has generated random and incomplete measures of leader performance. As an antidote to this haphazard approach, I have created a model (see exhibit 20.1) that evaluates and predicts performance using the components of a leader's persona and background.

This whole-person model rests on the premise that a leader's performance is affected by all of the conditions surrounding the individual, not just by selected aspects. The model's five components (which tie to the concepts discussed in this book) are made up of the traits and conditions that research, conducted over the past decades, has indicated to be contributors to effective performance:

1. *Values.* This component relates to a leader's fundamental beliefs and motivations. The values presented in this book

Exhibit 20.1 The Whole-Person Evaluation Model

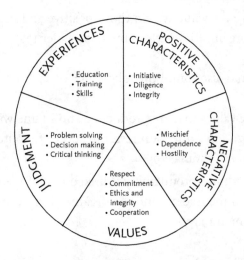

are supported by the literature (e.g., Bentz 1990; Conger and Kanungo 1990; Hallam and Campbell 1992; Hogan and Lock 1995; Hogan and Hogan 1994; Lombardo, Ruderman, and McCauley 1988; Lorr, Youniss, and Stefic 1991). I think of values in terms of the question, "Where do you want to go?"

2. *Positive characteristics.* This component includes characteristics—such as initiative, diligence, and integrity—that facilitate the leader's ability to get along and get ahead in the workplace. Such traits enable a person to abide by his values (Hogan 1992; Kets de Vries and Miller 1986). I think of positive characteristics in terms of the question, "What do you do to get there?"

3. *Negative characteristics.* This component comprises qualities—such as mischief, dependence, and hostility— that derail or inhibit a leader's personal and professional pursuits. Typically, negative characteristics create a distance between a person and everything else, making

her values difficult to share with and spread to others and causing low performance outcomes. I think of negative characteristics in terms of the question, "What do you do to get in the way of where you want to go?"

4. *Judgment.* This component describes the leader's cognitive process, including approaches to problem solving, decision making, and critical analysis. Judgment is the cross point between intelligence and personal style, in that it comes from a person's intellect, values, and personality. This unique combination is why two smart people faced with the same problem use different strategies and come up with different solutions. I think of judgment in terms of the question, "How do you solve problems along the way?"

5. *Experiences.* This component includes skills, education, training, background, history, and other personal and professional achievements and experiences that influence the leader's work. After understanding the strengths and barriers to leadership values in the first four areas, leaders can map their experiences to develop the leadership characteristics needed to drive values.

> The field of leadership is presently in a state of ferment and confusion. Most of the theories are beset with conceptual weaknesses and lack strong empirical support. . . . The confused state . . . can be attributed in large part to the disparity of approaches, the narrow focus of most researchers, and the absence of broad theories to integrate findings from the different approaches.
>
> —Gary Yukl and David Van Fleet (1992)

Each of the five components of the model should be examined to determine how well or how poorly a leader will perform. Research by the JDL Group significantly indicates that conflicts between any two or more areas (e.g., valuing helping others but having the negative characteristic of being harsh) will result in poor value and culture attainment. Understanding each area, and the combinations among them, results in exponential understanding of values above and beyond a single viewpoint.

VALUES AS THE KEYSTONE OF LEADER EFFECTIVENESS

Values, as illustrated in exhibit 20.1, represent only 20 percent of a leader's whole persona. So, you may ask, why write an entire book that extols the virtue of values? The answer is simple: Research shows that a leader's effectiveness starts with and is sustained by her value system. Consider these findings:

- Leader effectiveness entails convincing others to put aside their own self-interests to work on common goals that will lead to positive outcomes (Lock 1997).
- A leader's personal value system is ingrained, was solidified early in life, and will continue to be a factor throughout his career (Dawis 1980).
- Leaders inherently look for organizations that share their values or that otherwise stoke their motivations and give them the best opportunity to live their values (Schneider 1987). For example, the value of helping others is supported and shared by a hospital that provides appropriate and high-quality care to anyone regardless of the person's ability to pay.
- A leader actively promotes organizational behaviors and activities that enhance her own value system (Lock 1996).

Leaders have a tendency (often unconscious) to be attentive to areas that serve their own interests, but they give mostly lip service to other areas that do not present opportunities for fulfilling their values. Subordinates watch their immediate leader (not the CEO or the mission statement) to see what areas the leader focuses on. The subordinates then mimic the leader's emphasis (Pollak and Weiner 1995). Given a leader's heavy influence on her direct reports, the leader's values must be in line with the organization's mission, vision, and values. Otherwise, counterproductive performance may ensue (Lock 1997). Research on leader values further shows these:

- Employees stay with or leave an organization (or the immediate leader) on the basis of how well their focus or interests align with those of their leader (Doyle 1992). This alignment strengthens group identity and is thus beneficial to the organization, assuming that the shared focus (a) serves the organizational vision and goals and (b) leads to greater performance.

- Employee goal orientation is the most important contributor to how the team organizes itself and performs its organizational role (Hogan, Curphy, and Hogan 1994).

- Team effectiveness is directly related to the degree to which the team's and the organization's values and goals are similar (Meglino, Ravlin, and Adkins 1989).

In addition, research by the JDL Group shows that values (which are distinct from personality and other traits) are the keystone of leader effectiveness. That is, values stabilize and strengthen performance, which in turn becomes a model for others to emulate.

The Link Between Human Needs and Values

Values are evolutionary in nature and stem from people's basic social needs—namely, to get along with others, to get ahead in our pursuits, and to create order in our lives (personal and professional). Everyone has all three of these social needs, although the significance we give to each need varies, depending on our inherent values. For example, convicted corporate criminals, such as Bernie Madoff and Jeffrey Skilling, have a high need to get ahead but a low need to get along. Conversely, pacifists, such as Mother Teresa, have a high need to get along and low need to get ahead.

These social needs are automatic, ingrained, and largely unchanging. We create our own value system (with a personality that follows) to enable us to meet our needs. For example, a leader will build trust (a *value*) to fulfill her *need* to create order in her organization.

Exhibit 20.2 categorizes the values discussed in this book according to the three social needs.

Note that people's ability to make choices can cause the formation of *negative values.* Negative values are those that do not help us meet our basic social needs. For example, a leader who uses his position and power for personal gain idealizes self-interest and greed (negative values), which do not serve his needs for getting along, getting ahead, and creating order.

The Link Between Values and Leadership

As suggested by the research cited earlier, a leader's values often mirror (and, over time, could eclipse) organizational values. Organizational values then reflect what the leader wants, how she wants to treat and be treated by others, and what activities and interests she would like to pursue.

Exhibit 20.3 provides a framework for understanding how the components of the whole-person model (see exhibit 20.1) are affected by the leader's values.

Exhibit 20.2 Three Social Needs That Underlie Values

To Get Along	To Get Ahead	To Create Order
Respect	Commitment	Emotional intelligence
Cooperation and sharing	Ethics and integrity	Cohesiveness and collaboration
Conflict management	Desire to make a change	Trust
Servant leadership		Ethics and integrity
Interpersonal connection		

1. *Positive and negative characteristics.* These two components live in everyone's value system. A leader develops characteristics to influence others to work in ways that enhance his values. Positive traits can facilitate this attempt, while negative traits may hinder it.

2. *Judgment.* This component—the leader's thought process—is values based. Although a leader's problem-solving and decision-making styles are grounded in personality characteristics, her analytical abilities are driven by her values and needs. In evaluating alternatives and outcomes, she will weigh which option or result best suits the organizational values. Positive or negative personality traits also play a role in the leader's decision making. The

---

Exhibit 20.3 Values at the Core

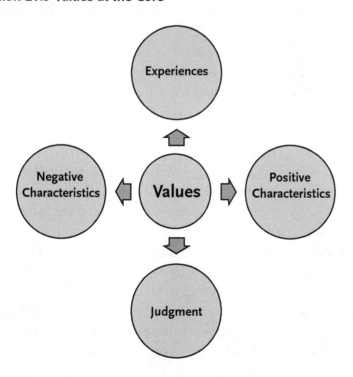

---

leader will use her judgment to assess the characteristics that get her closest to fulfilling her values.

3. *Experiences.* A leader's values regarding the experience component (e.g., lifelong learning, cross-training, workplace diversity) drive the initiatives pursued by the organization. When the organization changes its course (e.g., new boss, new vision) or no longer follows the values it shared with the leader, the leader separates from the organization and finds another with which to share his experience values.

For example, a leader who values respect develops an ambitious and outgoing trait. He sets lofty goals for himself and others, and he socializes with those who are in positions of power. In the process, he comes across as arrogant and as a social climber. Judging by the negative reaction to him, this leader's attempt to fulfill his value is one-sided.

Research by the JDL Group indicates that at least 50 percent of organizational leaders today display negative traits that cause stress, pressure, and poor performance among their employees. Although negative characteristics may deliver immediate results initially (e.g., bullies often get their way), these behaviors are not sustainable and are obstacles to achieving long-term values and needs.

Because positive and negative traits determine how well or poorly values and needs are met, successful leaders limit the negative and develop the positive. Having personal values that are in line with the organization's value system is great but is not enough; the leader's traits must also be aligned with these values. The JDL Group has shown that conflicts between traits and desired values are among the top areas of focus during interactions, costing healthcare organizations billions of dollars. For example, many healthcare executives value servant leadership and work commitment and ethics. But the personal traits they develop in pursuit of these values—such as aggressiveness and blind determination—can alienate their followers and discourage them from giving honest feedback to these leaders. As such, the leaders are confounded; they do not understand why their direct reports are distant despite their efforts to be "servants" to their work, staff, and organization.

Competencies and Behavior

Competencies and behaviors, although not specifically addressed by the whole-person model, are nonetheless associated with this approach.

Behaviors tend to be more myopic than the model itself. They are a person's individual actions that, when reviewed in total by others, define that person's personal characteristics or traits. In other words, behaviors represent the *why* and the *how* of a leader's performance. For instance, hand-wringing, hair flipping, and frowning are all behaviors associated with the characteristic or trait of anxiety. Competencies, on the other hand, are business-defined actions associated with several characteristics or traits represented across the model. In other words, competencies reflect *what* a person does on the job. For instance, when using the strategic orientation competency in the workplace, a leader will likely display characteristics associated with the judgment component (e.g., intelligent, analytical), the positive characteristics component (e.g., open to new ideas, takes initiative), and perhaps the negative characteristics component (e.g., arrogant, easily distracted). The combination of these characteristics in a leader leads to differential performance (as observed by others) on the competency.

SIX TENETS OF EVALUATING LEADER EFFECTIVENESS USING THE WHOLE-PERSON APPROACH

Assessing a leader's effectiveness is difficult in an environment over-run by thousands of performance measurement tools and theories.

The following tenets—specific to the whole-person approach—are intended to help leaders accurately understand, diagnose, and improve their own and their team's performance.

- *Tenet 1.* Performance measures should be well supported by research and should focus on the specific factors that drive effectiveness in your organization. The evaluation instruments (see the appendixes) presented in this book can provide a start.
- *Tenet 2.* One tool for each of the five components of the whole-person model should be identified. Typically, this identification entails examining various instruments and methods.
- *Tenet 3.* Performance data on all five components should be compiled into a single, easy-to-understand report. This custom content approach ensures that the data work to your advantage, not the other way around.
- *Tenet 4.* Assessments are the beginning of an improvement process, not the result. Accurate data and feedback force people to have direct, and even tough, conversations about their current inefficiencies. This discussion then leads to better outcomes.
- *Tenet 5.* Assessment should always go beyond the financial outcomes; it should include all five components of the whole-person model, including personal and organizational values. How and why the leader performs are just as important as the results she accomplishes.
- *Tenet 6.* Measuring the values and negative characteristics components takes creativity and diligence, given that the judgment and positive characteristics components make up about 95 percent of all available assessment tools.

A PRACTICAL EXAMPLE FOR IMPLEMENTING
THE WHOLE-PERSON APPROACH

This section is a step-by-step guide to applying to the workplace the concepts in this chapter and the values discussed in the book. The intent here is to show the clear connection between theory and practice; as such, this example could be used for teaching, discussion, and exercise purposes.

The work steps presented here are basic, but they lead to a better understanding of leadership effectiveness. Organizations that want to maximize their leaders' values-based effectiveness dig more deeply than this basic example allows, using well-validated measures of the five components of the whole-person model and creating detailed evaluations of leader performance.

Step 1: Define the corporate values. Most organizations have already completed this activity. If not, a quick survey of leaders is in order (e.g., "What are the top five values of our organization?"). Typically, a healthcare organization has at least three common values:

1. *Excellence.* We are committed to achieving the best service quality and using only best-practice solutions.
2. *People.* We respect coworkers, patients, and others in our community and are committed to open communication and teamwork.
3. *Service.* We strive to exceed the expectations and standards of those we serve by consistently providing the highest quality care.

Step 2: Pair each corporate value to leader values. In many instances, corporate and leader values align. Here is example grid A using the values espoused in this book:

Example Grid A

	Leader Values		
Corporate Values	To Get Along (Social Need)	To Get Ahead (Social Need)	To Create Order (Social Need)
Excellence	• Cooperation and sharing	• Commitment	• Ethics and integrity
People	• Respect in stewardship • Interpersonal connection		• Cohesiveness and collaboration • Trust
Service	• Servant leadership	• Desire to make a change	• Emotional intelligence

When matching corporate and leader values, the model will tend to show holes—that is, some leader values (categorized by social need) are not associated with corporate values. For example, in example grid A, the corporate value People is not associated with the leader value under To Get Ahead. These gaps should be seen as an opportunity for discussion on how to better align corporate and leader values and why such holes exist.

If one of the identified leader values is not used with any of the corporate values, is that acceptable? Is it expected? Why is it not important for the organization? Does the organization need to change anything?

Step 3: Tie each leader value to the other four components (experience, judgment, positive characteristics, negative characteristics) of the whole-person model. Use words that make sense to your organization, and provide specific characteristics instead of broad competencies. See example grid A.

Practical Exercise 1: Using example grid A as a format, fill out the people and service corporate values based on your experiences.

Practical Exercise 2: Take your organization's values statement and complete the exercise for your organization. Where are the holes in your model? Are all of the leadership values used? Are some values used in almost all corporate values and others in just a few? Is that acceptable? Have this discussion with someone in your organization (or your classmates), and evaluate what you have learned and how well you completed your grid.

Step 4: Tie each leader value to specific corporate effectiveness, competencies, or outcomes. Use words that make sense to your organization; making the model easy to understand is even more important than making it technically or scientifically accurate. For this step, ask the following questions for each component:

- *Experiences.* What organizational activities would a leader need to experience to test and validate the leader's willingness to follow this value?

- *Judgment.* If a leader shares this value, what would her decision-making style be? How would the leader solve problems? Would she focus more on data, processes, or people when making decisions?

- *Positive characteristics.* What characteristics does a leader need to perform these activities? How would I describe a leader with this value? Think of a leader who lives by this value, and describe that leader. Place your answers in a grid such as example grid A.

- *Negative characteristics.* What characteristics would "deep-six" a leader with respect to this value? If a leader is under stress and pressure, what poor characteristics would we see? Think of a leader who does not share each of the three corporate values (see step 1), and describe that leader. Place your answers in a grid such as example grid A.

- *Effectiveness, outcomes, or competencies.* We use these three labels interchangeably so as not to limit creativity. If a leader successfully lives by this value, what would the financial impact be to this part of the organization? How would it affect the people in the organization? How would it affect the patients? If the leader did not follow this value, how would it negatively affect the organization? If a leader lived this value, how would others describe the leader?

Only one of the three corporate values (excellence) is illustrated in the following example grid B, which brings up a few points:

1.   Example grid B is broad, completed with one- and two-word explanations, and not inclusive of all associated information. Your own grid should be as detailed as possible to enable you to effectively see and understand your organization's and leaders' performance expectations and their impact on the organization.

2.   The experience component is not included in example grid B. However, note that a multitude of experiences can indicate value acceptance, and experiences tend to be defined after the fact—that is, when the leader needs to learn how to espouse the value in his work group.

Example Grid B

Corporate Values	Leader Values	Positive Characteristics	Negative Characteristics	Judgment	Effectiveness/ Outcomes/ Competencies
Excellence	• Cooperation and sharing • Commitment • Ethics and integrity	• Outgoing • Ambitious • Conscientious • Sensitive • Learning oriented • Persistent	• Distrustful • Selfish • Mischievous • Inconsistent	• Considers data as well as experiences • Evaluates plans for accuracy • Follows data results	• Continuously implements new processes as information is received • Ranks in the top 90 percent on all key customer-excellence ratings • Has high team ratings • Institutes zero-complaint goal
People	• Respect in stewardship • Interpersonal connection • Cohesiveness and collaboration • Trust				
Service	• Servant leadership • Desire to make a change • Emotional intelligence				

Step 5: Evaluate a leader's effectiveness by following example grid B. Start at the effectiveness, outcomes, and competencies side, beginning with the far-right column and then filling in the middle of the grid. The reason for this order is that most people are better at first identifying *what* performance or outcome they desire before determining *how* it should be accomplished.

Next, think about the leader being evaluated and highlight the effectiveness, outcomes, and competencies; judgment; positive and negative characteristics; and values that this leader displays. Leave the rest unhighlighted. This step will serve as the basis of a performance discussion. How does the leader stack up? Compare the highlighted with the unhighlighted items. What characteristics are not highlighted? Are these the reasons the leader is not living up to expectations? Think of situations wherein the leader's deficiency (or presence of a negative characteristic) inhibited her from succeeding. What would you recommend to help the leader improve?

Step 6: Schedule a conversation with the leader. Explain the model, and discuss your findings. The leader should be actively involved in this conversation, offering comments, asking questions, and suggesting ideas for improvement.

CONCLUSION

I hope this chapter helps you understand the following points. First, leadership is not a "test of this" or a "list of that." Instead, it is a holistic understanding of how a person motivates others to put aside their own self-interests to work on group goals. Second, leaders drive their cultures, and—despite what is in the mission statement—subordinates look to their leaders' actions and behaviors to understand how to respond to workplace instances and interactions. Finally, while I recommend outside help to understand how to drive culture through leadership, leaders who self-reflect and know themselves well can purposefully and independently use the tools in this chapter to understand work direction and how to drive values through their own leadership style.

REFERENCES

Bentz, J. 1990. "Contextual Issues in Predicting High-Level Leadership Performance." In *Measures of Leadership*, edited by K. Clark and M. Clark, 131–43. West Orange, NJ: Leadership Library of America.

Borman, W., and S. Motowidlo. 1993. "Expanding the Criterion Domain." In *Personnel Selection in Organizations*, edited by N. Schmitt, W. Borman, and Associates, 71–98. San Francisco: Jossey-Bass.

Conger, J., and R. Kanungo. 1990. "A Behavioral Attribute Measure." Paper presented at the annual meeting of the Academy of Management, San Francisco.

Dawis, R. V. 1980. "Measuring Interests." *New Directions in Testing and Measurement* 7: 77–91.

Doyle, R. J. 1992. "Caution: Self-Directed Work Teams." *HR Magazine* 37 (6): 153–54.

Effron, M. 2014. "Start with the Science, Please!" *Insights*. Talent Strategy Group. Published June 14. http://talentstrategy group1.com/wp-content/uploads/2013/11/Start-with-the-Science-reduced.pdf.

Guzzo, R., and G. Shea. 1992. "Group Performance and Intergroup Relations." In *Handbook of Industrial and Organizational Psychology Volume 3*, 2nd ed., edited by M. Dunnette and L. Hough, 269–313. Palo Alto, CA: Consulting Psychologists Press.

Hackman, J. 1987. "The Design of Work Teams." In *Handbook of Organizational Behavior*, edited by J. Lorsch, 315–41. Englewood Cliffs, NJ: Prentice Hall.

Hallam, G., and D. Campbell. 1992. "Selecting Team Members." Paper presented at the annual meeting of the Society of Industrial and Organizational Psychology, Montreal, Quebec, Canada.

Hogan, J., and J. Lock. 1995. "A Taxonomy of Interpersonal Skills." Paper presented at the "Beyond Technical Requirements for Job Performance" symposium, conference of the Society for Industrial and Organizational Psychology, Orlando, Florida.

Hogan, R. 1992. "Personality and Personality Measurement." In *Handbook of Industrial and Organizational Psychology Volume 2*, 2nd ed., edited by D. Dunnette and L. Hough, 873–919. Palo Alto, CA: Consulting Psychologists Press.

Hogan, R., and R. Blake. 1996. "Vocational Interests." In *Behavior in Organizations*, edited by K. Murphy, 89–114. San Francisco: Jossey-Bass.

Hogan, R., G. Curphy, and J. Hogan. 1994. "What We Know About Leadership." *American Psychologist* 49 (6): 493–504.

Hogan, R., and J. Hogan. 1994. "The Mask of Integrity." In *Citizen Espionage: Studies in Trust and Betrayal*, edited by T. Sarbin, R. Carney, and C. Eoyang, 107–25. Westport, CT: Praeger.

Kets de Vries, M., and D. Miller. 1986. "Personality, Culture, and Organization." *Academy of Management Review* 11 (2): 266–79.

Kouzes, J. M., and B. Z. Posner. 2001. *The Leadership Challenge: How to Get Extraordinary Things Done in Organizations*, 5th ed. San Francisco: Jossey-Bass.

Lock, J. 1997. "The Relationship Between Trust and Leader–Group Processes." Paper presented at the "Personality Applications in the Workplace: Thinking Outside the Dots" symposium, 12th annual conference of the Society for Industrial and Organizational Psychology, St. Louis, Missouri.

———. 1996. "Developing an Integrative Model of Leadership." PhD diss., University of Tulsa, Oklahoma.

Lock, J., and L. Thomas. 1998. "The Effects of Leaders' Values on Group Citizenship." Poster presented at the 13th annual conference of the Society for Industrial and Organizational Psychology, Dallas, Texas.

Lombardo, M., M. Ruderman, and C. McCauley. 1988. "Explanations of Success and Derailment in Upper-Level Management Positions." *Journal of Business and Psychology* 2 (3): 199–216.

Lorr, M., R. Youniss, and R. Stefic. 1991. "An Inventory of Social Skills." *Journal of Personality Assessment* 57 (3): 506–20.

Manz, C., and H. Sims. 1987. "Leading Workers to Lead Themselves." *Administrative Science Quarterly* 32 (1): 106–28.

Meglino, B., E. Ravlin, and C. Adkins. 1989. "A Work Values Approach." *Journal of Applied Psychology* 74 (3): 424–32.

Pollak, R., and S. Weiner. 1995. "Team Assessment System: Factors of Team Effectiveness." Poster session presented at the conference of the Society for Industrial and Organizational Psychology, Orlando, Florida.

Schneider, B. 1987. "The People Make the Place." *Personnel Psychology* 40 (3): 437–53.

Yukl, G., and D. Van Fleet. 1992. "Theory and Research on Leadership in Organizations." In *Handbook of Industrial and Organizational Psychology Volume 3*, 2nd ed., edited by M. Dunnette and L. Hough, 147–97. Palo Alto, CA: Consulting Psychologists Press.

CHAPTER 21

The Need for Leaders

Christy Harris Lemak, PhD, FACHE

WE NEED LEADERS in healthcare. While our field has always presented unique and difficult challenges for managing and leading, the current and future landscape may be the most challenging yet. To achieve goals of better care, lower costs, improved patient experience, and improved community health, we need new types of leaders and new ways of developing them. We need leaders at all levels, coming from many different perspectives, and we need to improve the ways we develop leaders.

WE NEED TO RECOGNIZE AND FOSTER FRONTLINE LEADERS

All too often we think of leadership as something found in the C-suite or only among those who wear business suits. In fact, some of the best hospitals and health systems have discovered that the most important and influential leaders are found wearing scrubs or business casual attire at the front lines. These individuals, such as nurse supervisors and other clinical managers, may have received little or no leadership training but can be instrumental in shaping culture and transforming care delivery, improving the patient experience, and achieving needed cost reductions and quality improvements.

High-performing hospitals—such as those who have received the Malcolm Baldrige Award and others that are working toward high reliability—can demonstrate that frontline leaders are as important (or more important) than those in the C-suite (Griffith 2015; Griffith and White 2016). Their hospital leaders know and understand that developing human capital is a strategic imperative. Leaders must be able to develop others and create organizations that focus on developing leadership skills, not just in the executive suite.

As many hospitals and health systems invest time and money in quality improvement training, a disconnect sometimes emerges between training for improving patient care and training for managing caregivers and those who lead them. Great organizations reward and recognize leaders who develop other leaders at all levels. We need leaders who create great places to get care *and* great places to give care.

WE NEED TRANSFORMATIONAL LEADERS

The baby boomer generation that has led much of healthcare over the past decades is rapidly retiring. A growing gap in leadership talent can be found at many organizations. Emerging leaders need to step up to the challenge. In many cases, baby boomer leaders used more traditional, command-and-control approaches that were effective in the past but fall short as new generations of workers and new external challenges arise. Many members of the next generation are currently working in the field and may need support and leadership development to ascend into the C-suite.

Modern approaches to leadership involve moving beyond transaction-based and command-and-control leadership models toward transformational or servant leadership approaches in which leaders give individual consideration to the needs of followers (Greenleaf 2002; Kouzes and Posner 2012). Transformational leaders work to inspire, energize, and intellectually stimulate employees. Where command and control focused on hierarchy, transformational focuses on a greater shared purpose (e.g., putting patients first). As current CEOs retire, the next generation may need to seek out coaching, leadership development, and other training. The opportunity awaits. We need transformational leaders.

WE NEED LEADERS WHO CAN LEAD ACROSS COMMUNITIES

Leading to improve population health requires leaders from a variety of organizations to work together. For example, a hospital may need to collaborate with the local health department, federally qualified health centers, and volunteer organizations to adequately address readmission challenges and link underserved patients with medical homes and other needed services. Unfortunately, many hospital and health system leaders did not learn how to collaborate in graduate programs or medical schools. Until recently, graduate health administration programs were focused on teaching leaders to compete—to gain market advantage; to negotiate successfully with insurance companies; and to win the recruitment race for the best doctors, nurses, and management talent. To succeed in an environment of global commerce and bundled payments and to achieve organizational missions to improve the health of our communities, new skills and leadership approaches are critical.

Recent studies have shown that successful community-wide collaborations require skilled leadership, mutual respect and understanding among partner organizations, shared vision, common goals, and extensive relationships and communication linkages (Mattessich and Rausch 2014). Often, hospital executives do not recognize the existing status gaps and general lack of trust that may exist when working with other types of organizations in the community. Clinics that serve the uninsured and social service agencies may have tried to work with the local hospital in the past, but they found their calls were not answered or they were treated as "less important" by the relatively resource-rich hospital. Health system executives may be accustomed to giving directions and moving forward in styles that imply the input of others is unwelcome. Collaboration requires leaders to invest time to build trust, to engage multiple stakeholders, and to design and implement successful programs (Hansen 2009).

One program that serves the South Side of Chicago, the Medical Home Network (www.mhnchicago.org/index.html), was working to help coordinate and improve care for low-income women and families. The program required CEOs of various collaborating organizations—large hospitals, federally qualified health centers, the state Medicaid program, and others—to attend monthly meetings. This attendance was unusual because most of the organizations were accustomed to assigning such programs to vice presidents or others (not the CEO). In the required meetings, the executives began to collectively define the issues facing the uninsured and underinsured, to clearly see how each type of organization faced challenges, and to build respect and trust—all of which resulted in a successful, sustained set of innovative approaches to the complex challenges facing their communities.

We need leaders who can "check their organizational identity at the door" and work across their communities (often alongside their competitors) to create more coordinated care, to engage populations, and to improve the health of patients and the community.

WE NEED DIVERSE LEADERSHIP TEAMS

At front lines and across communities, we need diverse leadership teams. Population health improvement involves sustaining all members of the community at their highest possible levels of functioning, both for their individual happiness and for the collective community benefit (Kindig 2016). Improving population health is not just knowing and measuring but also making measurable improvements.

Leaders who understand these concepts and can bring together individuals and organizations may not be the leaders and leadership teams in US hospitals today.

We need leaders who can work with different types of organizations and build trust. We also need leaders who look like the communities served. Unfortunately, we now experience a pronounced lack of diversity in healthcare leadership teams and have seen very little change in the past few decades. Disparities in race and gender exist in hospital C-suites and boardrooms. To get to where we want to go, we need to enhance the commitment and capacity of healthcare systems and organizations to build and support engaged leadership teams that effectively understand and respond to the health needs of their communities in measurable and significant ways (Lemak, Paris, and McDonagh 2016). These teams need to understand community health needs and design solutions, and then implement them inside and outside the hospital walls.

Leadership equity can be defined as the intentional cultivation and strategic inclusion of diverse leaders in health system management and governance (Lemak, Paris, and McDonagh 2016). Recent studies indicate a large gender disparity in the hospital CEO role—a gap that has gotten bigger over the past decade (American College of Healthcare Executives [ACHE] 2012; 2013). The data are even more troubling when you consider race and ethnicity (ACHE 2015). Our C-suites and boardrooms are remarkably devoid of African Americans, Latinos, Muslims, and other minority populations, even as these groups are growing in many communities.

Organizations without leaders who reflect the makeup of their communities may be less likely to fully understand community needs, barriers to access, ways of improving healthy behaviors, and other important aspects of improving population health. Further, these differences often reflect long-standing community divides. It takes strong leaders working together to build trust and engage with citizens to overcome the difficult challenges we face today and tomorrow.

WHERE DO LEADERS IN HEALTHCARE COME FROM?

How can we improve our leadership pipeline and the ways we develop leaders? We focus on two main sources of healthcare leaders: graduate programs in healthcare leadership and healthcare organizations.

Graduate Programs in Health Administration

Since the late 1990s, graduate programs in health administration have focused on developing leadership skills using competency-based curricula. Many programs now emphasize experiential learning, self- and other-assessment of student leadership skills, and other ways of providing important knowledge, but they also focus on developing leadership skills. The efforts toward competency-based curricula and leadership have, in many ways, revolutionized graduate healthcare management education.

What can be done to improve how students learn in graduate school? Programs that focus on the individual strengths of students and provide opportunities for learning to "meet the student where she is" may see better results. In other words, a single, one-size-fits-all approach to learning will no longer work for graduate programs. Further, programs that maintain a robust, ongoing dialogue with the field of practice—through alumni boards, visiting executives, and the use of executives as teachers—may be better able to stay abreast of current trends in the field, in leadership needs, and in contemporary leadership development approaches.

Students who are given more frequent opportunities to learn in situ—that is, to do class projects in healthcare organizations, to gain in-depth internship or other field experiences, and to develop ongoing mentoring and coaching relationships with those in the field—may develop faster and achieve career success sooner. We need educational opportunities that develop leaders in the field, alongside current exemplar leaders.

Hospital and Healthcare Systems

Over the past 15 years, healthcare systems have begun to invest more in leadership development activities (Anderson and Garman 2014; Griffith and White 2016). Many are viewing human capital as their most improvable asset and one that is critical to achieving and sustaining organizational success. Many of these organizations—such as the Cleveland Clinic, Henry Ford Health System, and Stanford Medicine—have developed extensive leadership academies, with course catalogs of leadership development activities that are coordinated and sequenced to meet the various and evolving development needs of their employees.

Some large healthcare systems have well-developed "high potential" programs in which leadership talent is assessed annually and those with the potential for growth are given additional training, assigned coaches and sponsors, and carefully developed throughout increasing levels of responsibility in the organization (Anderson and Garman 2014; see the National Center for Healthcare Leadership [NCHL] website at www.nchl.org for more information). For example, the Penn Medicine Academy's Emerging Leaders Program identifies managers who show strong performance and potential and gives these emerging leaders opportunities to enhance their skills, preparing them for the next leadership role in the organization and beyond.

Another strategic human capital strategy used by some high-performing organizations is coaching. Organizations develop and deploy a team of trained and experienced coaches who work with top executives and those with high potential to build leadership skills on the job. In some cases, coaches work with leadership teams—not just at the C-suite but at other levels as well—to support team functioning and success. Cone Health, for example, uses coaches and tools both inside the system and by contract with outside coaches and programs. Other organizations that may not have the bandwidth to support internal coaches hire them from outside or create unique, team-based leadership development experiences facilitated by local experts.

For some organizations, leadership academies, team-development programs, and succession planning efforts provide a strategic perspective and frame for building new skills (such as collaboration) and tackling specific challenges (such as increasing diversity and inclusion). For example, members of the NCHL's Leadership Excellence Networks Diversity and Inclusion Council have (1) developed and distributed new tools for training leaders in the area of unconscious bias in hiring and promotion, (2) created guides for mentors, and (3) shared resources across their organizations. These and other organizations can closely link leadership development activities to organizational performance. They also find that they become magnets for top talent, as emerging leaders now seek environments where they can succeed immediately and where their leadership development is supported over time.

While many organizations are finding these human capital strategies to be effective, others—often smaller, independent hospitals—continue to identify succession planning as something they can improve on over the next several years (ACHE 2014). In short, for hospitals and health systems to succeed, they must develop the leaders they have, leveraging the human capital in the organization.

Academia and Practice Together

One opportunity for identifying and growing leaders may be in the magic that happens when academia and practice work more closely together.

One example is improving the administrative fellowship experience. High-performing organizations and others offer these one- or two-year experiences for new graduates with master of health administration degrees. For many organizations, such programs are a primary vehicle for identifying and recruiting new leaders (ACHE 2016). Recent efforts to improve fellowships themselves and the process by which organizations recruit participants include the National Council on Administrative Fellowships (http://nchl.

org/static.asp?path=2851,6549). This collective of academic program leaders and fellowship site leaders from across the country is working to establish and share best practices for the fellowship experience and to make applying for fellowships easier. Every hospital can and should reach out to the graduate programs in its area to begin a dialogue about how they might work together to develop leaders—from internship opportunities, to the administrative fellowship, to dedicated leadership training for mid- and senior-level leaders. For example, the University of Alabama at Birmingham's Department of Health Services Administration has developed customized programs that provide management training and quality and safety training for the managers and leaders at the University of Alabama at Birmingham Health System. Other programs provide management and leadership education for members of their hospital association or chapters of ACHE, the Healthcare Financial Management Association, and the Medical Group Management Association.

New efforts are also underway to bring the field of practice together with faculty members who are working to build the evidence base for healthcare management practice. One national program is called the Center for Healthcare Organizational Transformation (CHOT). In this National Science Foundation–sponsored effort, partners such as hospitals, health systems, and information technology vendors come together with disciplinary experts in engineering, management, and leadership to solve "wicked" healthcare problems together. Other, more localized efforts also succeed—as healthcare organizations and systems recognize the value of partnering with researchers in their local market to solve current challenges. Working together brings enhanced understanding of both perspectives. Scholars can then bring real-world experience into the classroom. Hospital leaders can bring the latest knowledge into their work, resulting in more evidence-based decision making. Partnerships across these previous silos are yielding some exciting gains in organizational performance and the knowledge and experience of current and emerging leaders.

Leaders in the field have an opportunity to invite faculty and students into their organizations to research, network, and learn. We can learn and work—together.

CONCLUSION

The need for excellent leaders in healthcare may be greater than ever, but so are the many opportunities to identify and develop capable leaders for the field. The complementary shifts to competency-based education and human capital approaches create the sense that we are moving in the right direction. We recognize that healthcare leadership is driven by values, and we are finding innovative ways to bring values into our work—in universities, boardrooms, and C-suites and, in the best cases, together.

We are working in many ways to develop transformational leaders who acknowledge that it will take all of us—collaboratively and collectively—to understand community needs, to inspire and energize associates inside and outside our organizations' walls, and to deploy strategies that we may not now imagine to improve the health of communities one patient at a time. From my perspective, the opportunities outweigh the potential obstacles by far. Let's do this—together.

REFERENCES

American College of Healthcare Executives (ACHE). 2016. "Postgraduate Fellowships: Creating Future Leaders." Accessed May 11. www.ache.org/postgrad/splash.cfm.

———. 2015. *A Racial/Ethnic Comparison of the Career Attainments in Healthcare Management.* Published January. www.ache.org/pubs/research/2014-Race-Ethnicity-Report.pdf.

———. 2014. *How Senior Leadership Teams Are Changing: A Survey of Freestanding Community Hospital CEOs.* Published Fall. www.ache.org/pubs/research/pdf/CEO-White-Paper-2014. pdf.

———. 2013. *Do Strategies That Organizations Use to Promote Gender Diversity Make a Difference?* Published Fall. www.ache. org/pubs/research/pdf/CEO_White_Paper_2013.pdf.

———. 2012. *A Comparison of the Career Attainments of Men and Women Healthcare Executives.* Published December. www. ache.org/pubs/research/2012-Gender-ExecSummary.pdf.

Anderson, M. M., and A. N. Garman. 2014. *Leadership Development in Healthcare Systems: Toward an Evidence-Based Approach.* National Center for Healthcare Leadership. Accessed May 11, 2016. http://nchl.org/Documents/Ctrl_Hyperlink/NCHL_ Leadership_Survey_White_Paper_Final_05.14_ uid6232014300422.pdf.

Greenleaf, R. K. 2002. *Servant Leadership: A Journey into the Nature of Legitimate Power and Greatness*, 25th anniversary ed., edited by L. C. Spears. New York: Paulist Press.

Griffith, J. R. 2015. "Understanding High-Reliability Organizations: Are Baldrige Winners Models?" *Journal of Healthcare Management* 60 (1): 44–62.

Griffith, J. R., and K. R. White. 2016. *The Well-Managed Healthcare Organization*, 8th ed. Chicago: Health Administration Press.

Hansen, M. T. 2009. *Collaboration: How Leaders Avoid the Traps, Create Unity, and Reap Big Results.* Boston: Harvard Business School Publishing.

Kindig, D. A (ed.). 2016. "What Is Population Health?" University of Wisconsin Population Health Sciences. Accessed

February 1. www.improvingpopulationhealth.org/blog/what-is-population-health.html.

Kouzes, J. M., and B. Z. Posner. 2012. *The Leadership Challenge: How to Make Extraordinary Things Happen in Organizations*, 5th ed. San Francisco: Jossey-Bass.

Lemak, C. H., N. Paris, and K. McDonagh. 2016. "Population Health Improvement Through Leadership Excellence." Presentation at the American College of Healthcare Executives Congress on Healthcare Leadership, Chicago, March.

Mattessich, P. W., and E. J. Rausch. 2014. "Cross-Sector Collaboration to Improve Community Health: A View of the Current Landscape." *Health Affairs* 33 (11): 1968–74.

CHAPTER 22

Does Leadership Matter?

Patrick D. Shay, PhD

BECKY AND ROB, two case managers at a small community hospital, have seen a lot in the past two years. Since their hospital was acquired by a large regional health system a couple years ago, they have witnessed considerable changes in their organization's workforce, policies, culture, and leadership, including the dismissal of their facility's long-tenured CEO, Walt Graham, and the introduction of a new CEO, Angela Gorski, who has a very different way of running things. In turn, they've also started to see a shift in the way their director of case management, Vivian Vargas, has approached her work. As they sit down to share lunch one day, these recent changes come up as the topic of conversation.

BECKY. Wow, it's been a rough day already. I saw Angela chewing out Vivian again today and thumping a big stack of reports that she seems extremely upset about. I'm not sure how long Vivian can keep putting up with this.

ROB. Yeah, she does seem to be under a lot of pressure now from Angela. I know Angela's always talking to her about those reports she gets from the corporate office. Of course, we feel the pressure too. Vivian seems different from how she used to be before the acquisition. She's much more impatient and stressed out now.

BECKY. Can you blame her? I'm glad I don't have to work directly for Angela. She seems so demanding and angry, and I'm not sure anyone can meet her expectations. I miss Walt. He knew how to treat people.

ROB. Walt certainly was easier to work for, I'll give you that. But I think he really struggled to motivate people, and he seemed to care more about being a friend than keeping anyone accountable around here. Walt was nice, but I don't think he was a very effective leader.

BECKY. Well, I certainly wouldn't call Angela an effective leader either. You can't be a leader and treat people so poorly.

ROB. I don't know. She does have to make tough decisions, and she seems to be trying hard to light a fire under everyone. Maybe it's just a different style of leadership?

BECKY. I doubt it. I mean, the hospital still seems to be struggling with the same problems we had before we got acquired. If what Angela's doing is leadership, does leadership even really matter?

THROUGHOUT THIS BOOK, the values and skills that characterize effective leaders have been convincingly presented and discussed, highlighting the importance of values-based leadership in today's complex and dynamic healthcare field. Yet reflecting on how these values and skills connect with their own personal experiences, some readers may question to what degree positive values and leadership skills indeed matter. Do we see leaders who exhibit such qualities truly realize success, and do leaders who fail to adhere to these values fail to realize desired performance levels?

Our nation's history is marked by individuals who led high-performing organizations yet failed to embody values such as integrity, trust, compassion, or respectful stewardship. We see this in popular culture as well, with an abundance of examples of unsavory organizational leaders depicted in film and television, from Mr. Potter in *It's a Wonderful Life* to Mr. Burns in *The Simpsons* to Bill Lumbergh in *Office Space*. Of course, the frustrations surrounding the seeming success of those who treat others poorly are not new to modern society; Job, the biblical figure, famously lamented the prosperity of the wicked amid his own suffering. In the same way, we are often challenged to reconcile those instances in which a leader can seemingly enjoy success while behaving badly.

On the other hand, many of us can think of leaders who embody the values and characteristics described in this book but who have not enjoyed success. Despite being admired and adored leaders, their organizations, departments, or units have failed to meet performance expectations. This outcome begs the question: Is there a connection between leaders' adoption and adherence to these values and effective performance? Or do leaders merely serve as figureheads, and do their skills and characteristics have little effect on organizational outcomes? Simply put, does leadership really matter?

To address these questions, this chapter looks at the extensive work of organizational researchers who have studied the role of leadership in organizations. We begin by considering the value of organization theory, followed by an examination of different perspectives in organization theory on the part leadership plays in organizational phenomena. The chapter concludes with a review of the academic literature on the connection between leadership and healthcare organizational performance.

ORGANIZATION THEORY

Although it may seem an unappealing exercise reserved for scholars stuck in an ivory tower, organization theory offers important insights and considerable value for today's healthcare leaders. More than just an academic discipline, organization theory serves as a tool that allows us to better make sense of complex phenomena, helping to simply explain and rationalize what we observe and experience in reality. Organization theory has been compared to looking through different sets of lenses, allowing us to clearly define and describe healthcare organizations to better understand what makes them effective, to make sense of the activities and behaviors that occur in them, and to predict organizational outcomes (Flood and Fennell 1995). In other words, engaging with organization theory provides value for anyone—practitioners and academics alike—interested in healthcare organizations. Shortell and Kaluzny (1988, 6) describe organization theory as a "*sine qua non* of modern healthcare management," recognizing that as we gain an understanding of different perspectives in organization theory, we can apply those models to the context of organizations, employees, teams, behaviors, environments, systems, and phenomena relevant to healthcare.

Scholars recognize that organizational phenomena occur at varying levels. As individuals and groups behave and work in an organizational setting, their personalities, activities, and other qualities affect the characteristics and outcomes of the overall organization. Theory that focuses on such phenomena among individuals and groups in organizations addresses the micro level of analysis, which is commonly referred to as *organizational behavior*. On the other hand, these individuals and groups make up entire organizations, and organizational characteristics, properties, activities, and dynamics in turn influence outcomes as well as the behaviors and actions of individuals. This attention to organizations as a whole and the activities that occur at organizational and interorganizational levels represents the macro level of analysis, also referred to simply as *organization theory*.

Micro and macro levels of analysis in organization theory speak to the role of leadership in organizational phenomena. Both levels include a variety of perspectives with different approaches to explaining the role of leaders. We now briefly summarize and address some of these perspectives.

Macrolevel Perspectives and Leadership

The modern canon of macrolevel organization theory includes a collection of perspectives that have emerged and developed since the mid-twentieth century, corresponding with the development and adoption of an open systems view of organizations (Mick and Shay 2014). This view was groundbreaking in its recognition that "organizations are not closed systems, sealed off from their environments" in the ways they can behave and operate independent of external circumstances and phenomena; instead, it argued that "environments shape, support, and infiltrate organizations," which must account for external factors, stakeholders, and phenomena to survive (Scott and Davis 2007, 31). Within this open systems approach, a diverse range of influential perspectives, such as contingency theory, transaction cost economics, resource dependence theory, and institutional theory, among others—have emerged and developed over the past 50 years.

Among these diverse perspectives, organization theorists have recognized the contrasting views regarding the role of leaders in directing organizational changes, shaping organizational life, and ultimately guiding organizational performance and survival. On one side of the debate, perspectives such as strategic management theory and social network theory are described as voluntaristic, depicting leaders as proactive and effective agents of change in their organizations (Abatecola 2012). For example, strategic management theory developed in part as a response to alternative perspectives that had offered limited views of managers' agency or organizations' adaptive abilities, instead emphasizing the role that leaders play in crafting organizational strategies in changing and complex environments so that the leaders may realize sustained competitive advantage (Hoskisson et al. 2011). Similarly, transaction cost economics is often summarized as suggesting organizational leaders face a "make or buy" decision. That is, leaders are viewed as integral to calculating and managing costs effectively in their decisions to either pursue integration strategies or engage in market exchanges for specific product lines or services (Tadelis and Williamson 2012). Perspectives that fall in the voluntaristic category implicitly—and at times explicitly—point to the notion that leadership indeed does matter. Leadership serves as one of the numerous building blocks on which organizational change occurs, influencing organizational performance and adaptation in tandem with other factors such as environmental characteristics, external relationships, competitive markets, and industry trends.

On the other side of the debate, perspectives such as population ecology and contingency theory have been described as deterministic in their views, assuming that leaders are limited in their abilities to drive organizational change. This approach instead emphasizes the role played by environmental forces and structural constraints that, in effect, determine organizational outcomes (Abatecola 2012). For example, population ecologists suggest that organizations are limited in their ability to adapt because of structural inertia, in such a way that sunk costs, limited information, political constraints, legal barriers, and organizational norms restrict the influence leadership may have on an organization's responses to environmental change (Salimath and Jones 2015). Similarly, some view contingency theory as implicitly suggesting that leaders have limited discretion over adopting an organizational structure that fits environmental and task contingencies (Van de Ven et al. 2012). Readers focusing on these and other deterministic perspectives may take such criticisms as evidence that these views portray leadership as largely ineffective when it comes to shaping organizational activities or outcomes.

However, despite this seeming divide among organization theorists, scholars caution that the deterministic perspective should not be misinterpreted as suggesting that leadership simply does not matter (Tolbert and Hall 2009). As Baum and Amburgey (2002, 305) argue, the deterministic approach to viewing the role of individuals in organizations might be more appropriately labeled as *probabilism* when contrasted with voluntarism, noting determinism's underlying recognition that "individuals do matter" but at the same time face severe constraints, affecting the probability that their actions can "consistently conceive and implement changes that improve organizational success and survival chances." A careful examination of classic works from deterministic perspectives helps reinforce this sentiment.

For example, Lawrence and Lorsch (1967, 242–45), in their seminal text that coined the term *contingency theory*, point to leadership as a critical component of organizational life, serving to infuse "purpose and meaning" in the organization, to formulate organizational strategies and goals, to "provide direction to the enterprise," and to assume a variety of roles such as driving innovation, integrating organizational components, and designing organizational forms. In their introduction of resource dependence theory, Pfeffer and Salancik (1978) note the constraints faced by organizational leaders and suggest that individual leaders play a restricted role in deciding organizational outcomes, but they simultaneously affirm the value of the leader's role in helping to reduce or remove constraints, manipulate environments, process external demands, and serve as an external symbol of the organization. Although population ecology views environments, rather than leaders, as "the driving force underlying organizational change" in specific circumstances, it "does not deny the importance of leaders," recognizing their ability to infuse organizational strategies and activities with purpose as well as the power of their decisions "in shaping organizational structures and processes" (Aldrich 1979, 22–23).

In sum, despite some popular misconceptions, macrolevel organization theory illustrates a common conviction among organization theorists and researchers that leadership indeed does matter. These varied perspectives account for the differing points of emphasis in recognizing the numerous factors that influence organizational activity and outcomes, including leadership. Macrolevel organization theory views leaders as actors who guide their organizations, shape organizational culture, navigate the external environment, and serve as agents of change to varying degrees. To examine theory-based views of leadership from individual- and team-based levels, we now turn to consider the literature on leadership from organizational behavior scholars.

Microlevel Perspectives and Leadership

Whereas macrolevel perspectives have approached the topic of leadership by asking what role leaders play in shaping organizational structures, activities, strategies, and performance, microlevel perspectives have instead asked what characterizes effective leaders. Over the past century, organizational scholars have developed a broad collection of theories that differentiate leaders from nonleaders and from one another, and these theories are often grouped into common categories: trait theories, behavioral theories, contingency theories, and contemporary theories.

Trait theories mark the early research efforts of leadership scholars, who originally assumed that leadership was innate, not taught (often referred to as the great man theory; see also chapter 2), and who sought to identify the specific traits of leaders (Hoffman et al. 2011). Although the search for a definitive list of traits that describe effective leaders initially generated much attention among researchers, early reviews by Stogdill (1948) and Mann (1959) raised doubts that leadership could be distilled to represent the possession of a specific combination of universal traits; as a result, many organizational scholars grew to view trait theories of leadership as too limited and simplistic. However, even in his influential work that questions whether a person with specific traits could effectively lead across different situations, Stogdill (1948, 65) also challenges his audience to avoid assuming "that leadership is entirely incidental, haphazard, and unpredictable," pointing to an underlying sentiment that leadership does matter.

As scholars turned away from trait theories in the mid-twentieth century, their attention was directed instead toward the behaviors that characterized effective leadership. Behavioral theories of leadership developed under the assumption that leadership skills could be taught, with some of the most recognizable behavioral theory research, including the studies developed at Ohio State University and the University of Michigan. These efforts have divided leadership behaviors into two categories: those behaviors that focus on tasks and production and those behaviors that focus on people and relationships. More recently, researchers have also studied change-oriented behaviors, which promote change, foster innovation, and inspire a vision for the future (DeRue et al. 2011). Collectively, the extant literature points to the influence of a leader's task, relational, and change-oriented behaviors on her own effectiveness as a leader as well as her group's performance (DeRue et al. 2011; Judge, Piccolo, and Ilies 2004). In this sense, we see that, once again, the work of organizational scholars suggests that leadership indeed matters.

Not long after the development of behavioral theories of leadership, numerous organizational scholars challenged the notion that a leader's effectiveness was solely determined by her behaviors or traits, leading to the emergence of contingency theories of leadership. These perspectives suggest that, more than just a leader's traits or behaviors, the *fit* between a leader's style and situational variables—including tasks, methods, and subordinate characteristics—influences performance (Robbins and Judge 2017). Widely recognized theories in this literature include Fiedler's (1967) contingency model of leadership effectiveness, House's (1971) path-goal theory of leadership, Hersey and Blanchard's (1972) situational leadership theory, and Graen and colleagues' (1973) leader–member exchange theory. These theories point to situations, relationships, and scenarios in which certain leadership behaviors, traits, and tactics may be more effective than others. Although this thinking has led some to suggest that, in certain instances, leaders' behaviors are irrelevant, this idea has been countered by those who suggest that contingency theories of leadership prove the value of leaders who can recognize the situations and contexts in which specific leadership approaches may be more or less appropriate (Jermier 1996).

As organizational studies have progressed through different theories of leadership, scholars have gained a deeper appreciation for the roles that traits, behaviors, and situations play in determining a leader's effectiveness. Contemporary theories of leadership build on these past efforts while also emphasizing the complexity that is inherent in the role of leadership and the myriad factors that may affect the outcomes of leadership efforts. Leadership concepts such as transformational, charismatic, adaptive, authentic, collaborative, ethical, and servant, among others, have been developed and emphasized by contemporary leadership scholars, bringing attention to the ways in which leaders can inspire, empower, foster trust, align values, change culture, and promote their followers' development (Borkowski 2016). Furthermore, contemporary theories challenge the traditional focus of leadership studies on the individual leader, calling for recognition of the diverse array of mechanisms that influence leadership dynamics, including situational, subordinate, structural, organizational, and environmental factors. For example, complexity leadership theory describes leadership as "a complex interplay of many interacting forces," and it highlights ways in which leaders can manage these forces by exercising adaptive, enabling, and administrative leadership, thereby enhancing "the overall flexibility and effectiveness of the organization" (Uhl-Bien, Marion, and McKelvey 2007, 314).

Collectively, the extant literature offers a variety of perspectives on leadership in organizations, including the different views of the role leaders play, constraints that affect leadership, traits and behaviors that characterize effective leaders, preferred leadership approaches for specific situations, and complex mechanisms that influence leaders' decisions and performance. As organization theory has advanced to successively introduce, evaluate, and even synthesize these varied perspectives, scholars have gained a more nuanced view of leadership in organizations. At the same time, we see a common thread across these different approaches when it comes to assessing leadership in organizations: It matters. Organization theorists, despite their different perspectives and emphases, consistently point to the important role played by leaders, in turn affecting their organizations, the individuals they work with, and their external environment. Given such convictions in organization theory, we now turn to look at the empirical evidence of leadership's impact on organizational outcomes.

THE EVIDENCE ON LEADERSHIP

Many studies in general management literature have asked whether leadership makes a difference in organizational performance, generally finding that, although "there are many potential performance measures that could be related to leader differences," leadership relates to performance "to a substantial degree" (Thomas 1988, 399). Gilmartin and D'Aunno (2007, 402) describe reviews of leadership research that have been published over the past half-century, highlighting the "steadily mounting evidence that leadership can matter significantly in a range of individual and group-level outcomes," including performance. Such studies draw attention to the relationship between "good" leadership and desirable outcomes, ranging from satisfaction to productivity and from financial performance to organizational climate (Koene, Vogelaar, and Soeters 2002).

Furthermore, research points not only to the relationship between effective leaders and desirable organizational outcomes but also to a connection between poor leadership and poor performance, suggesting that leaders' failure to exercise effective leadership skills translates to failed organizational performance. For example, destructive leadership practices are associated with outcomes such as job dissatisfaction, negative attitudes toward the leader, counterproductive work behaviors, and negative performance (Schyns and Schilling 2013). Researchers also note that, although toxic leaders who display "dark traits" such as Machiavellianism, narcissism, or psychopathy may seem to flourish in certain circumstances for a given period, they "typically derail somewhere down the line" and "eventually fall from grace" (Furnham, Richards, and Paulhus 2013, 206). In sum, as research on the effects of leaders on organizational outcomes has progressed, scholars have begun to argue that the empirical evidence is clear: "Leaders often have a substantial impact" (O'Reilly et al. 2010, 104).

Yet despite evidence in the general management literature that supports the importance of leadership, one must not assume that such support applies directly to the healthcare field, as past research finds leaders' impact on organizational performance varies across different industries (Wasserman, Anand, and Nohria 2010). Gilmartin and D'Aunno (2007) highlight the importance of specifically examining leadership in healthcare, as healthcare leaders face a litany of challenges (e.g., powerful professional groups, variable and uncertain performance criteria, continual technological advancements, widespread uncertainty, conflicting demands from external stakeholders) that make the healthcare setting a fertile ground for leadership research and theory development. Thus, our question of the importance of leadership extends specifically to healthcare organizations: Does leadership matter in healthcare?

The answer to that question, similar to the evidence generated in general management literature, is "yes." We see evidence in healthcare-related studies pointing to the impact of leadership on a variety of organizational outcomes and phenomena. In a comprehensive review of healthcare leadership literature published between 1989 and 2005, Gilmartin and D'Aunno (2007, 387) find that "leadership is positively and significantly associated with individual work satisfaction, turnover, and performance." At a broader level, research shows that leadership also plays a critical role in healthcare organization strategies. For example, Kaissi and Begun (2008) examine the role of leadership in hospital strategic planning processes, finding a significant relationship between leadership's active involvement in strategic planning and financial performance.

Healthcare in the twenty-first century has been characterized in part by an increased emphasis on quality of care and safety, which have emerged as chief concerns of healthcare providers today. Once again, empirical evidence suggests that leaders play a key role in their organizations' realization of quality and safety outcomes. A review by Singer, Benzer, and Hamdan (2015, 91) evaluates the role of collective learning in improving quality and safety in healthcare organizations, and their findings highlight "the importance of leadership in both promoting a supportive learning environment and implementing learning processes." Harrison and Coppola (2007) find evidence that hospital quality is positively related to hospital efficiency, and they argue this indicates that hospital leadership, by efficiently allocating resources and implementing effective work processes, can contribute to quality improvement across the organization. Furthermore, studies consistently point to a relationship between effective nursing leadership and various measures of quality and safety, such as improved patient satisfaction, reduced medication errors, and lower patient mortality (Wong, Cummings, and Ducharme 2013). Scholars emphasize the key role leadership plays in influencing an organizational climate that either promotes a patient safety culture—creating an "environment of psychological safety"—or invokes fear and blame in the event of errors, leading to a punitive atmosphere and "organizational silence and underreporting of error" (Henriksen and Dayton 2006, 1548). As Edmondson (2004, ii6) notes, variation in healthcare organizations' cultures, including patient safety culture, "is primarily driven by local leadership behavior."

Healthcare today is also characterized by growing emphases on team-based care and innovation, and the extant literature sees both topics as critical areas in which effective leadership can make a difference. For example, in a study of how healthcare leaders promote and facilitate team innovation in multidisciplinary care teams, West and colleagues (2003) observe that teams that had established and agreed on clear leadership roles achieved higher levels of performance and innovation. Researchers also note that leadership in healthcare organizations is not reserved for those individuals occupying formal administrative or management positions. They point to the importance of leadership provided by doctors, nurses, and other clinicians in the healthcare workforce, as "effective clinical leadership is associated with optimal hospital performance" and patient outcomes (Daly et al. 2014, 81). Similarly, O'Reilly and colleagues (2010, 111) make the important argument that organizational performance is not affected simply by the effectiveness of an individual senior leader but instead is determined through the aligned efforts of leaders at different levels of the healthcare organization.

CONCLUSION

This chapter began with a simple question: Does leadership matter? To address this question, we considered the varied perspectives on leadership offered in organization theory and then examined the extant evidence of the impact of leadership on organizational outcomes. Collectively, both organization theory and empirical evidence provide clear support for the important role leadership plays in organizational life, including healthcare organizations. However, the book is far from closed on the subject; we still require advances in organization theory and health services organization research to further our understanding of leadership in healthcare.

As we continue to gain a deeper appreciation for the multifaceted nature of leadership—as well as a deeper awareness of the intricate problems faced by our healthcare system—we will benefit from a continued exploration of the ways in which leaders and leadership practices affect individuals, groups, units, and healthcare organizations overall as well as the dynamics that allow leaders to most effectively overcome complex problems.

Does leadership matter? Yes, it does, and it is critically needed in our complex and fast-changing field as healthcare organizations seek to successfully meet today's myriad challenges to secure a better tomorrow.

REFERENCES

Abatecola, G. 2012. "Organizational Adaptation: An Update." *International Journal of Organizational Analysis* 20 (3): 274–93.

Aldrich, H. E. 1979. *Organizations and Environments.* Englewood Cliffs, NJ: Prentice Hall.

Baum, J. A. C., and T. L. Amburgey. 2002. "Organizational Ecology." In *The Blackwell Companion to Organizations,* edited by J. A. C. Baum, 304–26. Malden, MA: Blackwell Publishers.

Borkowski, N. 2016. *Organizational Behavior, Theory, and Design in Health Care,* 2nd ed. Burlington, MA: Jones & Bartlett Learning.

Daly, J., D. Jackson, J. Mannix, P. M. Davidson, and M. Hutchinson. 2014. "The Importance of Clinical Leadership in the Hospital Setting." *Journal of Healthcare Leadership* 6: 75–83.

DeRue, D. S., J. D. Nahrgang, N. Wellman, and S. E. Humphrey. 2011. "Trait and Behavioral Theories of Leadership: An Integration and Meta-Analytic Test of Their Relative Validity." *Personnel Psychology* 64 (1): 7–52.

Edmondson, A. C. 2004. "Learning from Failure in Health Care: Frequent Opportunities, Pervasive Barriers." *Quality and Safety in Health Care* 13 (suppl. 2): ii3–ii9.

Fiedler, F. E. 1967. *A Theory of Leadership Effectiveness.* New York: McGraw-Hill.

Flood, A. B., and M. L. Fennell. 1995. "Through the Lenses of Organizational Sociology: The Role of Organizational Theory and Research in Conceptualizing and Examining Our Health Care System." *Journal of Health and Social Behavior* special issue: 154–69.

Furnham, A., S. C. Richards, and D. L. Paulhus. 2013. "The Dark Triad of Personality: A 10 Year Review." *Social and Personality Psychology Compass* 7 (3): 199–216.

Gilmartin, M. J., and T. A. D'Aunno. 2007. "Leadership Research in Healthcare: A Review and Roadmap." *Academy of Management Annals* 1 (1): 387–438.

Graen, G., F. Dansereau Jr., T. Minami, and J. Cashman. 1973. "Leadership Behaviors as Cues to Performance Evaluation." *Academy of Management Journal* 16 (4): 611–23.

Harrison, J. P., and M. N. Coppola. 2007. "Is the Quality of Hospital Care a Function of Leadership?" *Health Care Manager* 26 (3): 263–72.

Henriksen, K., and E. Dayton. 2006. "Organizational Silence and Hidden Threats to Patient Safety." *Health Services Research* 41 (4, pt. 2): 1539–54.

Hersey, P., and K. H. Blanchard. 1972. *Management of Organizational Behavior: Utilizing Human Resources*. Englewood Cliffs, NJ: Prentice Hall.

Hoffman, B. J., D. J. Woehr, R. Maldagen-Youngjohn, and B. D. Lyons. 2011. "Great Man or Great Myth? A Quantitative Review of the Relationship Between Individual Differences and Leader Effectiveness." *Journal of Occupational and Organizational Psychology* 84 (2): 347–81.

Hoskisson, R. E., M. A. Hitt, W. P. Wan, and D. Yiu. 2011. "Antecedents and Precedents to Porter's *Competitive Strategy*." In *Competition, Competitive Advantage, and Clusters: The Ideas of Michael Porter*, edited by R. Huggins and H. Izushi, 57–73. New York: Oxford University Press.

House, R. J. 1971. "A Path Goal Theory of Leader Effectiveness." *Administrative Science Quarterly* 16 (3): 321–39.

Jermier, J. M. 1996. "The Path-Goal Theory of Leadership: A Subtextual Analysis." *Leadership Quarterly* 7 (3): 311–16.

Judge, T. A., R. F. Piccolo, and R. Ilies. 2004. "The Forgotten Ones? The Validity of Consideration and Initiating Structure in Leadership Research." *Journal of Applied Psychology* 89 (1): 36–51.

Kaissi, A. A., and J. W. Begun. 2008. "Strategic Planning Processes and Hospital Financial Performance." *Journal of Healthcare Management* 53 (3): 197–208.

Koene, B. A. S., A. L. W. Vogelaar, and J. L. Soeters. 2002. "Leadership Effects on Organizational Climate and Financial Performance: Local Leadership Effect in Chain Organizations." *Leadership Quarterly* 13 (3): 193–215.

Lawrence, P. R., and J. W. Lorsch. 1967. *Organizations and Environment: Managing Differentiation and Integration*. Boston: Division of Research, Graduate School of Business Administration, Harvard University.

Mann, R. D. 1959. "A Review of the Relationship Between Personality and Performance in Small Groups." *Psychological Bulletin* 56 (4): 241–70.

Mick, S. S. F., and P. D. Shay. 2014. *Advances in Health Care Organization Theory*, 2nd ed. San Francisco: Jossey-Bass.

O'Reilly, C. A., D. F. Caldwell, J. A. Chatman, M. Lapiz, and W. Self. 2010. "How Leadership Matters: The Effects of Leaders' Alignment on Strategy Implementation." *Leadership Quarterly* 21 (1): 104–13.

Pfeffer, J., and G. R. Salancik. 1978. *The External Control of Organizations: A Resource Dependence Perspective*. New York: Harper & Row.

Robbins, S. P., and T. A. Judge. 2017. *Organizational Behavior,* 17th ed. Boston: Pearson.

Salimath, M. S., and R. Jones III. 2015. "Population Ecology Theory: Implications for Sustainability." *Management Decision* 49 (6): 874–910.

Schyns, B., and J. Schilling. 2013. "How Bad Are the Effects of Bad Leaders? A Meta-analysis of Destructive Leadership and Its Outcomes." *Leadership Quarterly* 24 (1): 138–58.

Scott, W. R., and G. F. Davis. 2007. *Organizations and Organizing: Rational, Natural, and Open System Perspectives.* Upper Saddle River, NJ: Pearson Prentice Hall.

Shortell, S. M., and A. D. Kaluzny. 1988. *Health Care Management: A Text in Organization Theory and Behavior,* 2nd ed. New York: John Wiley & Sons.

Singer, S. J., J. K. Benzer, and S. U. Hamdan. 2015. "Improving Health Care Quality and Safety: The Role of Collective Learning." *Journal of Healthcare Leadership* 7: 91–107.

Stogdill, R. M. 1948. "Personal Factors Associated with Leadership: A Survey of the Literature." *Journal of Psychology* 25 (1): 35–71.

Tadelis, S., and O. E. Williamson. 2012. "Transaction Cost Economics." In *The Handbook of Organizational Economics,* edited by R. Gibbons and J. Roberts, 159–90. Princeton, NJ: Princeton University Press.

Thomas, A. B. 1988. "Does Leadership Make a Difference to Organizational Performance?" *Administrative Science Quarterly* 33 (3): 388–400.

Tolbert, P. S., and R. H. Hall. 2009. *Organizations: Structures, Processes, and Outcomes,* 10th ed. Upper Saddle River, NJ: Pearson Prentice Hall.

Uhl-Bien, M., R. Marion, and B. McKelvey. 2007. "Complexity Leadership Theory: Shifting Leadership from the Industrial Age to the Knowledge Era." *Leadership Quarterly* 18 (4): 298–318.

Van de Ven, A. H., R. Leung, J. P. Bechara, and K. Sun. 2012. "Changing Organizational Designs and Performance Frontiers." *Organization Science* 23 (4): 1055–76.

Wasserman, N., B. Anand, and N. Nohria. 2010. "When Does Leadership Matter? A Contingent Opportunities View of CEO Leadership." In *Handbook of Leadership Theory and Practice: A Harvard Business School Centennial Colloquium on Advancing Leadership,* edited by N. Nohria and R. Khurana, 27–64. Boston: Harvard Business Press.

West, M. A., C. S. Borrill, J. F. Dawson, F. Brodbeck, D. A. Shapiro, and B. Haward. 2003. "Leadership Clarity and Team Innovation in Health Care." *Leadership Quarterly* 14 (4–5): 393–410.

Wong, C. A., G. G. Cummings, and L. Ducharme. 2013. "The Relationship Between Nursing Leadership and Patient Outcomes: A Systematic Review Update." *Journal of Nursing Management* 21 (5): 709–24.

Professional and Personal Values Evaluation Form

OUR BEHAVIORS REVEAL our values more clearly than our words do. Civility often prevents us from saying what we truly think, but it does not always prevent us from reacting with our body. As a result, we give out two varying reactions to one scenario.

This questionnaire assesses your values on the basis of your perception and others' perceptions. It contains two tools—Self-Perception and Others' Perception.

Directions: After you complete the Self-Perception questionnaire, ask two to three fellow team members whom you think know you well to complete the Others' Perception questionnaire. Ideally, a neutral third party should collect the completed questionnaires and compile averages and ranges for the answers. This process might encourage others to be more honest when evaluating you. Following discussions with the neutral third party about the responses, you may meet with the individuals who evaluated you to compare and contrast all perceptions.

SELF-PERCEPTION OF VALUES

1. I respect other people.

Strongly Disagree	Disagree	Neither Disagree nor Agree	Agree	Strongly Agree
1	2	3	4	5

2. I serve as a good steward of the talent, authority, resources, and position I hold.

Strongly Disagree	Disagree	Neither Disagree nor Agree	Agree	Strongly Agree
1	2	3	4	5

3. I am an ethical person.

Strongly Disagree	Disagree	Neither Disagree nor Agree	Agree	Strongly Agree
1	2	3	4	5

4. I keep my word.

Strongly Disagree	Disagree	Neither Disagree nor Agree	Agree	Strongly Agree
1	2	3	4	5

5. I seek to develop positive and wholesome relationships with others.

Strongly Disagree	Disagree	Neither Disagree nor Agree	Agree	Strongly Agree
1	2	3	4	5

6. I desire to serve others.

Strongly Disagree	Disagree	Neither Disagree nor Agree	Agree	Strongly Agree
1	2	3	4	5

7. I want to make a difference and effect positive changes and contributions.

Strongly Disagree	Disagree	Neither Disagree nor Agree	Agree	Strongly Agree
1	2	3	4	5

8. I am committed to the vision and goals of my organization.

Strongly Disagree	Disagree	Neither Disagree nor Agree	Agree	Strongly Agree
1	2	3	4	5

9. I work hard.

Strongly Disagree	Disagree	Neither Disagree nor Agree	Agree	Strongly Agree
1	2	3	4	5

10. I am a highly dedicated person.

Strongly Disagree	Disagree	Neither Disagree nor Agree	Agree	Strongly Agree
1	2	3	4	5

11. I am emotionally mature.

Strongly Disagree	Disagree	Neither Disagree nor Agree	Agree	Strongly Agree
1	2	3	4	5

12. I value the contributions of a team.

Strongly Disagree	Disagree	Neither Disagree nor Agree	Agree	Strongly Agree
1	2	3	4	5

13. I cooperate with fellow team members.

Strongly Disagree	Disagree	Neither Disagree nor Agree	Agree	Strongly Agree
1	2	3	4	5

14. I share information and other resources with fellow team members.

Strongly Disagree	Disagree	Neither Disagree nor Agree	Agree	Strongly Agree
1	2	3	4	5

15. I try to build trust with others.

Strongly Disagree	Disagree	Neither Disagree nor Agree	Agree	Strongly Agree
1	2	3	4	5

16. I am willing to trust others.

Strongly Disagree	Disagree	Neither Disagree nor Agree	Agree	Strongly Agree
1	2	3	4	5

17. I affirmatively try to bring conflict to the surface to manage it effectively.

Strongly Disagree	Disagree	Neither Disagree nor Agree	Agree	Strongly Agree
1	2	3	4	5

OTHERS' PERCEPTION OF_____(Insert Name Here)_____'S VALUES

1. Your colleague respects other people.

Strongly Disagree	Disagree	Neither Disagree nor Agree	Agree	Strongly Agree
1	2	3	4	5

2. Your colleague serves as a good steward of the talent, authority, resources, and position she/he holds.

Strongly Disagree	Disagree	Neither Disagree nor Agree	Agree	Strongly Agree
1	2	3	4	5

3. Your colleague is an ethical person.

Strongly Disagree	Disagree	Neither Disagree nor Agree	Agree	Strongly Agree
1	2	3	4	5

4. Your colleague keeps her/his word.

Strongly Disagree	Disagree	Neither Disagree nor Agree	Agree	Strongly Agree
1	2	3	4	5

5. Your colleague seeks to develop positive and wholesome relationships with others.

Strongly Disagree	Disagree	Neither Disagree nor Agree	Agree	Strongly Agree
1	2	3	4	5

6. Your colleague desires to serve others.

Strongly Disagree	Disagree	Neither Disagree nor Agree	Agree	Strongly Agree
1	2	3	4	5

7. Your colleague wishes to make a difference and effect positive changes and contributions.

Strongly Disagree	Disagree	Neither Disagree nor Agree	Agree	Strongly Agree
1	2	3	4	5

8. Your colleague is committed to the vision and goals of your organization.

Strongly Disagree	Disagree	Neither Disagree nor Agree	Agree	Strongly Agree
1	2	3	4	5

9. Your colleague works hard.

Strongly Disagree	Disagree	Neither Disagree nor Agree	Agree	Strongly Agree
1	2	3	4	5

10. Your colleague is a highly dedicated person.

Strongly Disagree	Disagree	Neither Disagree nor Agree	Agree	Strongly Agree
1	2	3	4	5

11. Your colleague is emotionally mature.

Strongly Disagree	Disagree	Neither Disagree nor Agree	Agree	Strongly Agree
1	2	3	4	5

12. Your colleague values the contributions of a team.

Strongly Disagree	Disagree	Neither Disagree nor Agree	Agree	Strongly Agree
1	2	3	4	5

13. Your colleague cooperates with fellow team members.

Strongly Disagree	Disagree	Neither Disagree nor Agree	Agree	Strongly Agree
1	2	3	4	5

14. Your colleague shares information and other resources with fellow team members.

Strongly Disagree	Disagree	Neither Disagree nor Agree	Agree	Strongly Agree
1	2	3	4	5

15. Your colleague tries to build trust with others.

Strongly Disagree	Disagree	Neither Disagree nor Agree	Agree	Strongly Agree
1	2	3	4	5

16. Your colleague is willing to trust others.

Strongly Disagree	Disagree	Neither Disagree nor Agree	Agree	Strongly Agree
1	2	3	4	5

17. Your colleague affirmatively tries to bring conflict to the surface to manage it effectively.

Strongly Disagree	Disagree	Neither Disagree nor Agree	Agree	Strongly Agree
1	2	3	4	5

Emotional Intelligence
Evaluation Form

EMOTIONAL INTELLIGENCE IS a person's maturity quotient. Maturity is the ability to manage emotions, make sound decisions, positively influence others, and be self-aware. The questions in this instrument assess the emotional intelligence of a person in the workplace on the basis of the perception of those she/he works with directly or has worked with directly in the past.

Directions: Read each question carefully and circle the answer that most appropriately describes the person being evaluated. There are no right or wrong answers, but carefully reflect on each question and answer.

You have been asked to evaluate ___(insert name here)___ along several interpersonal dimensions. Five or more individuals—peers and subordinates—are completing this questionnaire. When you are finished, please return your questionnaire to ___(name of third party)___, who will compile the results and provide summary averages to the person named above. Because the questionnaire does not require your name, your participation is anonymous; please do not share your responses with anyone.

What is your relationship to the person being evaluated? Please check one.

_____ Peer (work at same organization)
_____ Peer (work elsewhere)
_____ Subordinate
_____ Superior (full-time paid boss)
_____ Superior (voluntary board member)
_____ Other

1. This leader creates the feeling that she/he looks forward to each day with positive anticipation.

Strongly Disagree	Disagree	Neither Disagree nor Agree	Agree	Strongly Agree
1	2	3	4	5

2. This leader truly believes that her/his work really makes a difference in her/his organization.

Strongly Disagree	Disagree	Neither Disagree nor Agree	Agree	Strongly Agree
1	2	3	4	5

3. This leader has an even temper.

Strongly Disagree	Disagree	Neither Disagree nor Agree	Agree	Strongly Agree
1	2	3	4	5

4. This leader rarely gets frustrated.

Strongly Disagree	Disagree	Neither Disagree nor Agree	Agree	Strongly Agree
1	2	3	4	5

5. This leader has the creative ability to solve problems among people.

Strongly Disagree	Disagree	Neither Disagree nor Agree	Agree	Strongly Agree
1	2	3	4	5

6. This leader truly enjoys being with other people.

Strongly Disagree	Disagree	Neither Disagree nor Agree	Agree	Strongly Agree
1	2	3	4	5

7. This leader has strong control over her/his emotions.

Strongly Disagree	Disagree	Neither Disagree nor Agree	Agree	Strongly Agree
1	2	3	4	5

8. When times get tough in the work setting, others can turn to this leader for guidance.

Strongly Disagree	Disagree	Neither Disagree nor Agree	Agree	Strongly Agree
1	2	3	4	5

9. When mistakes are made, this leader's first instinct is to take corrective action (rather than place blame).

Strongly Disagree	Disagree	Neither Disagree nor Agree	Agree	Strongly Agree
1	2	3	4	5

10. Other people would describe this leader as a person who does not "fall apart" under pressure.

Strongly Disagree	Disagree	Neither Disagree nor Agree	Agree	Strongly Agree
1	2	3	4	5

11. This leader is well suited for her/his career.

Strongly Disagree	Disagree	Neither Disagree nor Agree	Agree	Strongly Agree
1	2	3	4	5

12. If this leader had the chance to start her/his career all over again, she/he would still choose a leadership position.

Strongly Disagree	Disagree	Neither Disagree nor Agree	Agree	Strongly Agree
1	2	3	4	5

13. This leader respects other people.

Strongly Disagree	Disagree	Neither Disagree nor Agree	Agree	Strongly Agree
1	2	3	4	5

14. This leader is highly motivated.

Strongly Disagree	Disagree	Neither Disagree nor Agree	Agree	Strongly Agree
1	2	3	4	5

15. Others would say this leader has her/his ego under control.

Strongly Disagree	Disagree	Neither Disagree nor Agree	Agree	Strongly Agree
1	2	3	4	5

16. This leader has an appropriately high level of self-esteem.

Strongly Disagree	Disagree	Neither Disagree nor Agree	Agree	Strongly Agree
1	2	3	4	5

17. Although this leader may at times get upset or angry, she/he has the ability to control emotions.

Strongly Disagree	Disagree	Neither Disagree nor Agree	Agree	Strongly Agree
1	2	3	4	5

18. This leader has an appropriately high level of motivation.

Strongly Disagree	Disagree	Neither Disagree nor Agree	Agree	Strongly Agree
1	2	3	4	5

19. This leader always seeks win–win solutions in conflict situations.

Strongly Disagree	Disagree	Neither Disagree nor Agree	Agree	Strongly Agree
1	2	3	4	5

20. This leader would be the last person I would describe as a hopeless individual.

Strongly Disagree	Disagree	Neither Disagree nor Agree	Agree	Strongly Agree
1	2	3	4	5

21. Although impatient for positive results, this leader does not allow her/his impatience to create a negative working environment.

Strongly Disagree	Disagree	Neither Disagree nor Agree	Agree	Strongly Agree
1	2	3	4	5

22. This leader is a person whom others trust.

Strongly Disagree	Disagree	Neither Disagree nor Agree	Agree	Strongly Agree
1	2	3	4	5

23. This leader is appropriately self-confident without being overbearing.

Strongly Disagree	Disagree	Neither Disagree nor Agree	Agree	Strongly Agree
1	2	3	4	5

24. This leader is sensitive to others' feelings.

Strongly Disagree	Disagree	Neither Disagree nor Agree	Agree	Strongly Agree
1	2	3	4	5

25. This leader listens well.

Strongly Disagree	Disagree	Neither Disagree nor Agree	Agree	Strongly Agree
1	2	3	4	5

26. The last description you would expect to hear of this leader is "flies off the handle a lot."

Strongly Disagree	Disagree	Neither Disagree nor Agree	Agree	Strongly Agree
1	2	3	4	5

27. This leader maintains a good balance in life.

Strongly Disagree	Disagree	Neither Disagree nor Agree	Agree	Strongly Agree
1	2	3	4	5

28. This leader is emotionally stable and healthy.

Strongly Disagree	Disagree	Neither Disagree nor Agree	Agree	Strongly Agree
1	2	3	4	5

29. This leader faces setbacks and adversity well.

Strongly Disagree	Disagree	Neither Disagree nor Agree	Agree	Strongly Agree
1	2	3	4	5

30. This leader would not be described as hostile.

Strongly Disagree	Disagree	Neither Disagree nor Agree	Agree	Strongly Agree
1	2	3	4	5

31. This leader has developed good mechanisms to get feedback from others.

Strongly Disagree	Disagree	Neither Disagree nor Agree	Agree	Strongly Agree
1	2	3	4	5

Leadership Team Evaluation Form

ALTHOUGH THIS QUESTIONNAIRE has not been validated (i.e., no study has been performed to determine the correlation between the results of this questionnaire and performance outcome, such as profitability, patient satisfaction, physician satisfaction, or employee satisfaction), it provides the team with an initial tool for assessing the components of team effectiveness.

Because each component contributes to the overall efficiencies and inefficiencies of the team, each must be independently evaluated. To ensure comprehensive representation, all team members must complete the questionnaire. To ensure confidentiality of the responses, the team must select a neutral third party to collect the questionnaires; tally the ratings; and write a report, which must be distributed to the team for discussion.

Directions: Rate the following statements as correctly as possible. Please submit your completed questionnaire to _____(name of third party)_____ by __(date)__. Please do not share your responses with others.

TEAM LEADERSHIP

1. The CEO or leader is not autocratic.

Strongly Disagree	Disagree	Neither Disagree nor Agree	Agree	Strongly Agree
1	2	3	4	5

2. The CEO or leader does not make team decisions outside meetings.

Strongly Disagree	Disagree	Neither Disagree nor Agree	Agree	Strongly Agree
1	2	3	4	5

3. The CEO or leader develops an atmosphere that encourages openness.

Strongly Disagree	Disagree	Neither Disagree nor Agree	Agree	Strongly Agree
1	2	3	4	5

4. The CEO or leader is not afraid to be a full and equal participant in team processes.

Strongly Disagree	Disagree	Neither Disagree nor Agree	Agree	Strongly Agree
1	2	3	4	5

5. In establishing the team, the CEO or leader ensures that all team members understand the decisions that should be made within the team setting and the decisions that should be made outside the team setting.

Strongly Disagree	Disagree	Neither Disagree nor Agree	Agree	Strongly Agree
1	2	3	4	5

6. The CEO or leader ensures that time is set aside to occasionally discuss roles and decision-making rules and protocols.

Strongly Disagree	Disagree	Neither Disagree nor Agree	Agree	Strongly Agree
1	2	3	4	5

TEAM COMPATIBILITY

7. Members share common values and goals.

Strongly Disagree	Disagree	Neither Disagree nor Agree	Agree	Strongly Agree
1	2	3	4	5

8. Members have personal compatibility.

Strongly Disagree	Disagree	Neither Disagree nor Agree	Agree	Strongly Agree
1	2	3	4	5

9. Members have professional compatibility.

Strongly Disagree	Disagree	Neither Disagree nor Agree	Agree	Strongly Agree
1	2	3	4	5

TEAM INTERACTION

10. Members have camaraderie.

Strongly Disagree	Disagree	Neither Disagree nor Agree	Agree	Strongly Agree
1	2	3	4	5

11. Members occasionally socialize outside of the workplace.

Strongly Disagree	Disagree	Neither Disagree nor Agree	Agree	Strongly Agree
1	2	3	4	5

12. Members have frequent communication.

Strongly Disagree	Disagree	Neither Disagree nor Agree	Agree	Strongly Agree
1	2	3	4	5

13. Members have open and candid conversations.

Strongly Disagree	Disagree	Neither Disagree nor Agree	Agree	Strongly Agree
1	2	3	4	5

14. Members exchange accurate and timely information, prohibit or limit exaggeration, and discourage information hiding.

Strongly Disagree	Disagree	Neither Disagree nor Agree	Agree	Strongly Agree
1	2	3	4	5

TEAM MIND-SET AND STRUCTURE

15. Members are committed to the same goals.

Strongly Disagree	Disagree	Neither Disagree nor Agree	Agree	Strongly Agree
1	2	3	4	5

16. Each member understands her/his role within the team.

Strongly Disagree	Disagree	Neither Disagree nor Agree	Agree	Strongly Agree
1	2	3	4	5

17. Members have actively and openly discussed team roles.

Strongly Disagree	Disagree	Neither Disagree nor Agree	Agree	Strongly Agree
1	2	3	4	5

18. Members have mutually agreed to the assignment of team roles.

Strongly Disagree	Disagree	Neither Disagree nor Agree	Agree	Strongly Agree
1	2	3	4	5

19. Members are highly interdependent.

Strongly Disagree	Disagree	Neither Disagree nor Agree	Agree	Strongly Agree
1	2	3	4	5

20. The team has a high energy level.

Strongly Disagree	Disagree	Neither Disagree nor Agree	Agree	Strongly Agree
1	2	3	4	5

21. Members acknowledge, discuss, and manage conflict.

Strongly Disagree	Disagree	Neither Disagree nor Agree	Agree	Strongly Agree
1	2	3	4	5

22. Members are frank with each other and engage in little politics.

Strongly Disagree	Disagree	Neither Disagree nor Agree	Agree	Strongly Agree
1	2	3	4	5

23. The size of the team is between 6 and 11.

Strongly Disagree	Disagree	Neither Disagree nor Agree	Agree	Strongly Agree
1	2	3	4	5

24. There is a proper balance of titles among members.

Strongly Disagree	Disagree	Neither Disagree nor Agree	Agree	Strongly Agree
1	2	3	4	5

TEAM MEETINGS

25. Meetings are well organized.

Strongly Disagree	Disagree	Neither Disagree nor Agree	Agree	Strongly Agree
1	2	3	4	5

26. Meetings have objectives.

Strongly Disagree	Disagree	Neither Disagree nor Agree	Agree	Strongly Agree
1	2	3	4	5

27. The agenda is followed closely during meetings.

Strongly Disagree	Disagree	Neither Disagree nor Agree	Agree	Strongly Agree
1	2	3	4	5

28. Members show appropriate courtesy to each other during meetings.

Strongly Disagree	Disagree	Neither Disagree nor Agree	Agree	Strongly Agree
1	2	3	4	5

29. All members actively participate in meetings.

Strongly Disagree	Disagree	Neither Disagree nor Agree	Agree	Strongly Agree
1	2	3	4	5

30. Meetings have an appropriate level of formality but are not stiff.

Strongly Disagree	Disagree	Neither Disagree nor Agree	Agree	Strongly Agree
1	2	3	4	5

31. Meetings end with an understood conclusion.

Strongly Disagree	Disagree	Neither Disagree nor Agree	Agree	Strongly Agree
1	2	3	4	5

TEAM DECISIONS

32. The team observes decision-making protocols.

Strongly Disagree	Disagree	Neither Disagree nor Agree	Agree	Strongly Agree
1	2	3	4	5

33. The entire team is responsible for decision making.

Strongly Disagree	Disagree	Neither Disagree nor Agree	Agree	Strongly Agree
1	2	3	4	5

34. The entire team has been trained in decision-making techniques.

Strongly Disagree	Disagree	Neither Disagree nor Agree	Agree	Strongly Agree
1	2	3	4	5

35. The team has openly discussed its decision-making styles and processes.

Strongly Disagree	Disagree	Neither Disagree nor Agree	Agree	Strongly Agree
1	2	3	4	5

36. The entire team realizes the danger of using compromise as the only end result of a decision-making process.

Strongly Disagree	Disagree	Neither Disagree nor Agree	Agree	Strongly Agree
1	2	3	4	5

Grading Healthcare
Team Effectiveness

THE FOLLOWING ASSESSMENTS are meant in the spirit of continuous improvement. They follow the outline provided in chapter 18, "Evaluating Team Effectiveness." A review of that chapter can be helpful in better understanding the nature of this analysis. A fictional evaluation of a poorly performing team is presented here first. It is followed by a blank form for you to use in conducting a similar evaluation of your team.

SAMPLE LEADERSHIP TEAM: STRUCTURE
Size

The team comprises 20 or more individuals—far too large to be truly effective.

Grade = D–

Hierarchy

There is very little proper balance among the leadership team members. For a variety of reasons, some individuals simply carry more weight. As one CEO is known to say, "In some teams, you count votes, but in many others, you weigh the votes."

Grade = F

Membership

The senior team comprises some members whose position cannot possibly be linked to any logical reason to be a member.

Grade = C

SAMPLE LEADERSHIP TEAM: ACTIVITIES
Decision Making

The team has no defined rationale for decision making. Few team members have ever taken a course in decision making. The team members simply kick ideas around until the leader (usually the CEO) calls for a decision—or, worse yet, indicates her own decision.

Grade = D–

Meetings

Typical meetings are the source of wasted time, rudeness, passive-aggressive behavior, and frequent sneaky looks at the smartphone by all in attendance. Few meetings are well planned, and fewer still provide any logical flow regarding topics. Tactical matters compete with strategic matters, and most participants secretly view the entire event as an enormous time waster.

Grade = F

Necessity

The team has far too many meetings, and those it holds usually last far too long.

Grade = C–

Objectives, Agendas, and Handouts

Although agendas are used much more than in the past, the effectiveness stops there. Minutes are characteristically a huge waste of effort. The traditional rule requiring that handouts be provided in advance is among the most violated.

Grade = D

Roles and Norms

Roles are played and norms exist—but they are rarely, if ever, discussed.

Grade = D–

Time

"Talk, talk, talk, when do we eat?" Because the meetings are not managed in a timely manner, the team finds it must often order in for food when important and weighty topics are discussed (and of course, all topics are important and weighty for this team).

Grade = D

Format

The team has used the same meeting format for decades. They rarely mix up methods or approaches.

Grade = C

Etiquette

Smartphones, administrative assistants entering the room to pass notes to some higher-level team members, sidebar conversations, late arrivals, early departures, doodling, lots of talk but very little frankness, breaking up the flow of conversation by getting up for a coffee refill—have we said enough?

Grade = D–

Participation

Some members are highly participative, some rarely participate, and some fall in the middle. The team leader is rarely effective in using techniques to draw all members out. Moreover, the power imbalance means that much goes unsaid for fear of retribution.

Grade = C

Wrap-Up

The team does poorly in wrapping up its meetings. Although it has adopted some of the agenda-tracking minutes that are used in quality improvement work groups, the agendas are rarely followed.

Grade = C

Protocol Development

There are no set ground rules and guidelines for team interaction, meeting management, and decision making.

Grade = D

Hearing the Famous Statement

A vast majority of the time, the following statement can be heard at the end of the typical leadership meeting: "Meeting's over, let's get back to work."

Grade = A

YOUR TEAM: STRUCTURE
Size

Grade =

Hierarchy

Grade =

Membership

Grade =

YOUR TEAM: ACTIVITIES
Decision Making

Grade =

Meetings

Grade =

Necessity

Grade =

Objectives, Agendas, and Handouts

Grade =

Roles and Norms

Grade =

Time

Grade =

Format

Grade =

Etiquette

Grade =

Participation

Grade =

Wrap-Up

Grade =

Protocol Development

Grade =

Hearing the Famous Statement

Grade =

Index

Note: Italicized page locators refer to text in exhibits.

Reciprocity, 121–22
Recognition: of others, 126
Recruitment, 35, 82, 205–6
Reference checking, 116, 206
Resistance, 243
Resource dependence theory, 351
Respect: cases and exercises, 102–3; collaboration and, 95; others' definition of, 95–97; self-evaluation questions, 102; showing for others, *93*, 124; value of, 92, 101
Restless discontent, 157
Retirement planning, 306–7
Retreats, 193, 210, 242, 275
Risks, 162
"Road Not Taken, The" (Frost), 58, *59*
Rousseau, D. M., 48
Rubenstein, Maj. Gen. D., 244
Rylatt, A., 156

Sacrifices, 177–78
Safety outcomes, 357
Saks, A. M., 132
Salancik, G. R., 351
Salovey, P., 188
Santora, J. C., 60
Sarros, J. C., 60
Scholarly discourse, 49
Scientific management, 24
Self-awareness, 38, 99, 190–91
Self-centeredness: self-esteem *vs.*, 93–94, *94*
Self-esteem: self-centeredness *vs.*, 93–94, *94*
Self-evaluation, 293–308; continuing education, 298; personal mission statement, 295, *296*; personal/professional style, 295–97; questions, 308; values, 297; vignette, 293–94
Selfish behavior: minimizing, 223–24
Self-reflection, 193, 308, 330
Self-tributes, 307–8
Selling leadership style, 29
Senge, P., 140
Senior leaders: challenges encountered by, 79–80, *80*; organizational factors and, 80–85; self-evaluation questions, 86

Senior management: team code of conduct, *211*
Servant leaders: behaviors exhibited by, 141; skills of, 142–48
Servant leadership, 139–50, 334; cases and exercises, 149–50; goals of, 140; proponents of, 140; self-evaluation questions, 149; traditional leadership *vs.*, *141*; transformational leadership and, 142; vignette, 139–40
Setbacks, 195
7 Habits of Highly Successful People, The (Covey), 47, 181–82
Shared responsibility, 96
Shared vision: lack of, 85
Sharing, 68
Shortell, S. M., 269, 348
Singer, S. J., 357
Singh, K., 191
Situational leadership theory, 26, 28, 29, 38, *39*, 353
Six Sigma, 163
Skilling, J., 319
Skills-based leadership, 50
SMART goals, 161
Smiling: power of, 126–27
Social competence, 191
Social exchange theory, 237–38
Social needs, 319–20, *320*
Social network theory, 349
Sokolov, J. J., 38
SOPs. *See* Standard operating procedures (SOPs)
Sousa, M., 140
Span of control theory, 24
Staff: connection with, 147–48
Standard operating procedures (SOPs), 213
Stanford Medicine, 339
Start-and-stop hiring, 82
Steele, G. D., 291
Stogdill, R. M., 26, 32, 34, 352
Stogdill's Handbook of Leadership, 32
Strategic management theory, 349
Strengths-based leadership, 48
Strengths Based Leadership (Rath and Conchie), 48

About the Author

CARSON F. DYE, FACHE, president and CEO of Exceptional Leadership, LLC, is a seasoned leadership consultant with more than 40 years of leadership and management experience. Over the past 20 years, he has conducted hundreds of leadership searches for healthcare organizations, helping to fill chief executive officer, chief operating officer, chief financial officer, and physician executive roles in health systems, academic medical centers, universities, and freestanding hospitals.

Dye has provided clients with extensive counsel in succession planning, leadership assessment, CEO evaluation, coaching, and retreat facilitation. He is certified to use the Hogan Leadership Assessment tests for evaluation, coaching, and leadership development. He also has extensive experience working with physician leaders and has helped organizations establish physician leadership development programs.

Dye has served as an executive search consultant and partner with Witt/Kieffer, TMP Worldwide, and LAI/Lamalie Associates. Prior to these roles, he was partner and director of Findley Davies's healthcare consulting division in Toledo, Ohio. Dye has 20 years of experience in healthcare administration, serving in executive-level positions at St. Vincent Mercy Medical Center in Toledo, the Ohio State University Medical Center in Columbus, and Children's Hospital Medical Center and Clermont Mercy Hospital—both in Cincinnati.

Dye has been a regular faculty member for the American College of Healthcare Executives (ACHE) since 1987 and has presented workshops for 40 state and local hospital associations. He also teaches in the ACHE Board of Governors Examination preparation course. In addition, Dye is a faculty member of The Governance Institute and currently holds a faculty appointment at the University of Alabama at Birmingham in its executive MBA program.

Dye has written ten previous books, all with Health Administration Press, including two James A. Hamilton Book of the Year winners, *Developing Physician Leaders for Successful Clinical Integration* (2013) and *Leadership in Healthcare: Values at the Top* (2000). His other titles include *The Healthcare Leader's Guide to Actions, Awareness, and Perceptions*; *Exceptional Leadership: 16 Critical Competencies for Healthcare Executives*; *Winning the Talent War*; and *Protocols for Healthcare Executive Behavior*. The Dye–Garman Leadership Competency Model, found in *Exceptional Leadership*, has been used by many healthcare organizations as a competency model for assessment, executive selection, development, and succession planning. Dye earned his BA from Marietta College and his MBA from Xavier University.

About the Contributors

CHRISTY HARRIS LEMAK, PHD, FACHE, is professor and chair of the Department of Health Services Administration at the University of Alabama, Birmingham.

Dr. Lemak teaches and conducts scholarship in the areas of healthcare management and leadership development with an emphasis on how leadership and organizational factors can lead to high performance in healthcare.

Her research includes projects to examine (1) a complex pay-for-performance incentive program for physicians in Michigan and (2) the relationships among organizational culture, management practice, and surgical outcomes in a multihospital surgical collaborative. She is currently examining new ways of measuring hospital and system performance.

Dr. Lemak holds a PhD in health services organization and policy from the University of Michigan, MHA and MBA degrees from the University of Missouri at Columbia, and a BS in health planning and administration from the University of Illinois.

JARED D. LOCK, PHD, is a licensed industrial/organizational psychologist. He is founder of the JDL Group, an international assessment and consulting firm focused on maximizing productivity, and cofounder of Convergent, LLC, creator of the world's first change management software, which manages the complete life cycle of culture and change initiatives.

Prior to establishing his own organizations, Dr. Lock was director of consulting services at Hogan Assessment Systems. He was the lead Hogan consultant on executive-level selection and development, and he regularly partnered with organizational executives and boards on selection and development programs. With stints at both Sprint and Jeanneret & Associates, he has more than 15 years of healthcare industry experience. He has been the lead researcher on the development and validation of automated, multihurdle, multitechnique selection systems for many *Fortune* 100 organizations. Furthermore, he has created seven unique and proprietary assessments of job-specific performance for various clients throughout the world. In addition, he has been instrumental in implementing leadership development and succession planning programs for several *Fortune* 100 companies, and he has conducted a great deal of research on executive selection and performance.

Dr. Lock has written more than 60 book chapters, papers, and presentations. He holds a BA in psychology from the University of Kansas and an MA and a PhD in industrial/organizational psychology from the University of Tulsa.

Patrick D. Shay, PhD, is an assistant professor in the Department of Health Care Administration at Trinity University in San Antonio, Texas, where he teaches graduate courses on such topics as health services organization and policy, population health management, and healthcare organization theory and behavior. His research applies organization theory to healthcare organization phenomena, including the activities and configurations of local multihospital systems as well as the impact of regulation on post-acute care providers, among others. Prior to his doctoral studies, he worked as a healthcare administrator for a post-acute care system in south Texas.

Dr. Shay is a member of the American College of Healthcare Executives. He received his BS in business administration and MS in healthcare administration from Trinity University and his PhD in health services organization and research from Virginia Commonwealth University.